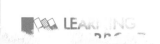
GATTEFOSSÉ'S AROMATHERAPY

Preface by Dr Foveau de Courmelles
Lauréat of the Académie de Médicine

Edited by Robert B. Tisserand

Translated by Louise Davies
in collaboration with
First Edition Translations Ltd

From the original French text
"Aromathérapie: Les Huiles essentielles
hormones végétales"
First published in 1937

SAFFRON WALDEN
THE C. W. DANIEL COMPANY LIMITED

Publisher's Acknowledgement

The publisher is grateful to
Miss Jeanne Rose, Miss Susan Knepper
and Miss Julie E. Johnson
for their help in acquiring an initial
draft translation of this work.

First published in France in 1937 by
Girardot & Cie, Paris

This English-language edition
First published in Great Britain in 1993 by
The C. W. Daniel Company Ltd
1 Church Path, Saffron Walden
Essex, CB10 1JP, England

Reprinted 1995

ISBN 0 85207 236 8

Designed by Peter Dolton
Designed and produced in association
with Book Production Consultants plc, Cambridge
Typeset by Rowland Phototypesetting Ltd,
Bury St Edmunds, Suffolk
Printed and bound in England by St Edmundsbury Press Ltd,
Bury St Edmunds, Suffolk

Contents

Frontispiece   iv

Editor's Introduction   v

Preface by Dr Foveau de Courmelles   vii

Foreword   xi

Chapter I   1
Human, Animal and Plant Smells

Chapter II   11
The Classification of Essential Oils

Chapter III   21
Essences in Ancient Pharmacopoeias

Chapter IV   37
More Recent Works on Essential Oils

Chapter V   55
Aromatherapy

Chapter VI   97
Tests on the Anti-Toxic Action of
Essential Oils

Conclusions   117

Bibliography   121

Biography   133

Works of R. M. Gattefossé   137

Notes   139

Index   149

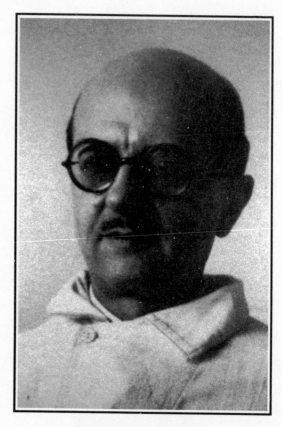

René-Maurice Gattefossé
1881–1950

Editor's Introduction

It has been a revelation and an immense pleasure to edit this English translation of the first book to be written on aromatherapy. After searching sporadically for it for 20 years I had begun to even doubt its existence until Ian Miller of The C. W. Daniel Company traced Gattefossé's son in France, and obtained a copy.

René-Maurice Gattefossé was not the first to use essential oils therapeutically, nor to write about such use, both events having taken place 1,000 years ago. However, he had an unprecedented vision. Not one of his predecessors, during the thousand years since the invention of distillation, had seen that the therapeutic application of essential oils constituted a discipline in its own right. A few had sometimes come close to it, and Gattefossé had many contemporaries who were engaged in aromatherapy research, but none of them seems to have possessed his pioneering enthusiasm for the subject. It was this vision and dedication which inspired him to coin the word "aromatherapy".

As a chemist Gattefossé was not a part of the natural therapy movement and he did not share the holistic, "alternative" approach to aromatherapy so prevalent today. Nevertheless he was fascinated by certain esoteric subjects, and wrote about psychic strength, Atlantis, and prehistoric metaphysics. He was clearly very perceptive, and many of his ideas (such as synergy, the psychological effects of fragrance, and percutaneous administration) have helped to form the framework of aromatherapy today.

Gattefossé knew his limitations. He knew that many of the questions he wrestled with would be resolved in time, and he makes frequent reference to the illustrious future in store for aromatherapy. He speaks of his pioneering work as "the dogged work of a chemist and perfumer who patiently endeavoured to prove the efficacy of fragrant substances". As a chemist he knew the importance of a chemical understanding of aromatherapy, and as a perfumer he perceived the psychotherapeutic benefits of fragrance itself. His chemical observations have been further developed in recent years by a dedicated group of French doctors. However they did not follow up on Gattefossé's psychotherapeutic insights which have been further developed by fragrance researchers and aromatherapists. That he recognised the importance of both approaches confirms the man's unrivalled stature. There can be no doubt that he did more than anyone to lay the foundations for aromatherapy this century.

With the benefits of hindsight and over 50 years of subsequent research it is all too easy to find fault with some of Gattefossé's conclusions. (For example, he felt that the terpenes found in essential oils were much more hazardous than we now know them to be.) His book, however, retains many strengths, notably its many case studies, or "observations" from doctors Forgues, Meurisse, Marchand and Sassard. In particular the antiseptic and healing powers of lavender oil on wounds cannot fail to impress even the most skeptical reader. Wound healing was a major problem, and the cause of many deaths during the First World War. Essential oils might have been more widely used during the Second World War if penicillin had not been discovered, but they were used to a limited degree – for instance some Australian troops carried tea tree oil, until supplies ran out.

This book represents a "missing link" for 20th century aromatherapy, a link between the 1890's and the 1990's. But it is much more than that, it is also the most important book because without it aromatherapy might never have happened.

Robert Tisserand
July 1992

PREFACE

Aromatherapy? A therapy or cure using aromas, aromatics, scents? Yes! They can all be therapeutic if used, dosed and administered correctly and at the right time. Animals, vegetables and minerals all produce aromas.

These curative properties are found mainly in plants, although certain animals, and humans too, should not be discounted. No longer is the idea of human radiation dismissed, since it is now even acknowledged that microbes produce emanations in mitogenesis.

Fragrances, and thus essential oils, play an important role in our lives. Fragrance attracts. Fragrances are diffused in the air in someone's honour. "Extracts" – perfume essences – are actually extracted or alternatively manufactured synthetically.

In bygone ages, pouring oil on someone's feet was a common way of showing respect. Throughout history, perfumes have also played an important role in religious practices. The world over, the bodies of important people were buried and covered in aromatics and fragrances.

People have different individual smells depending on their colour, race and homeland. And of course, some smells attract while others repel.

What are smells made of? How do they affect us? How do we extract them? Which are the best? The ones we prefer. It is said that "a wise man never discusses tastes and smells," yet there seems to be universal agreement about some of them.

These are the questions which R. M. Gattefossé, a chemist, has been studying for close on fifty years of dogged and patient work, and in which he has enlisted my support. Having worked in the physical and chemical laboratories of the science faculties as an electro-radiologist, and having paid dearly for it by being exposed to pervasive radiation, perfumes which do not seem to register much in terms of the electrical vibrations found everywhere and in everything – for all nature is scented – I feel unable to appreciate his work in full. I must therefore restrict my appraisal to his written work and his innovations. I could say that his work has the tempting aroma of knowledge, wisdom and utility. It is full of promise, has a heady bouquet and, although he has studied unpleasant smells, they do not filter through his erudite words to us. With the right knowledge, everything can be put to good use.

Man emits, gives off, radiates smells, he "odiferates", if I may take the liberty of creating a neologism. At times he can smell quite bad when he is ill, sick or unclean. In a crowd, he can smell even worse and, in this regard, Jean Jacques Rousseau wrote "Man is a poison to man". In a documented work entitled *Les odeurs du corps humain* [The odours of the human body], the late Dr E. Monin found that the smells exhaled by patients were an excellent diagnostic aid. It is often possible to smell fever or cancer in a sickroom.

Smells can charm and be health-giving, or quite the opposite. Our smells can attract or repel. They can be therapeutic, create sympathetic feelings or antipathies which sometimes impose themselves on our organisms and should not be disregarded. We often corrupt our instincts – just as we taint the air with our unpleasant smells – with poorly assimilated knowledge or, as Michelet said, with instruction or education. I would say that we make inadequate use of our senses and, with regard to smell, they play a major, sorely neglected role. In "Aromatherapy" one of our senses in particular, the sense of smell, makes the fullest use of scents in their simplest and most effective form, as revealed by Mr Gattefossé on many occasions.

Living beings, even plants, which provide so many odours and medicines, all seem to have a certain appreciation of smells and perfumes, and to react to them. A particular plant cannot thrive in particular surroundings, in a particular type of shade . . . A flower worn by one woman will wilt because of the efflux, the emanation from her body, whereas it will last well on another woman. A small insect has been found living with ants, which seems to have the role of scenting the home of these social and hard-working *Hymenoptera*. Is this a luxury – or a necessity?

Other insects flee from the perfumes of plants. *Datura stramonium*, a poisonous plant, wards off weevils and, in barns, wheat protected by the plant (which smells unpleasant to weevils) will be left alone, undamaged by them. This is why the first antiseptics used in medicine smelt rather unpleasant, with their carbolic acid base. I witnessed this at the time when Pasteur started his work and Lister and Lucas-Championnière put it into practice. Since then, just as pills are now "sugar-coated", antiseptics have been scented (but not at the cost of asepsis) and thymol[1] has enjoyed widespread use for some time now. In 1887, the late Professor Budin taught how to use this pleasant antiseptic – a plant extract, like so many others – in his obstetric work and operations. Plants often provided the active ingredient and the aroma used.

---

[1] Please refer to page 139 for Notes.

Today herbal medicine is popular, and rightly so, as are natural plant and mineral substances and, in this well-documented book, the reader will find a wide array of useful, applied, monitored, observed and accepted substances.

For instance, pine forests, with their smell of resin or turpentine, provide health-giving and fragrant volatile essences which penetrate our lungs and often have a beneficial effect. Sun and light promote their release and penetration, while altitude and proximity to the sea provide a different quality of air, frequently ozonised. The pervasive aromas are continually and repeatedly drawn into our lungs when we breathe, for we inhale at least half a litre sixteen times a minute. If we multiply these figures over 24 hours, the quantitative penetration of a scent and its effect on the organism become clear. Ozone, an electrically charged oxygen, which, according to patients, smells of sulphur, can, in comparison to that produced by an electrostatic machine (franklinisation) or faradic equipment, be charged, in a pine forest, with redolent vapours which contribute their own invigorating action on the lungs, although too much can cause congestion of the lungs. Ultraviolet rays increase ozone production and penetration.

Light, like so many physical forces, such as electricity and heat, can be and is actually absorbed into all substances exposed to it, put in contact with it and which can convey it. Many examples of this will be found in this work.

Mr Gattefossé believes that fragrant, volatile substances play the valuable role of anti-toxic and antiviral agents, being similar to vitamins and hormones. It is an imaginative theory – but altogether possible.

Interpenetration is fairly generalised in the natural world. This phenomenon, which, since 1911, I have called "integrated light", produces vitamins and bestows on those bodies containing them various vital properties of great importance which seem to reach their culmination in irradiated ergosterol. The property of absorbing fragrances is related to this. As we know, plants are all the more active when exposed to sunlight, that is, when gathered in bright sunshine. This is generally true – as tradition has it – because certain hours of the day or night bestow different properties on plants and their fragrances.

Knowledge of how smells are absorbed and incorporated is important because, to be effective, they must penetrate the skin. We know that skin is more porous to gases than to liquids and solids. Gases, and thus aromas – whether highly pervasive or not –

incorporated in glycerides, readily penetrate the skin where the blood can transport them. The choice of solvent depends on the particular application, while the substances and their roles are clearly defined by the author.

Numerous forms of application have also been developed, such as the extreme fragmentation of musk in the atmosphere, as it has therapeutic properties, like so many of the fragrances so closely studied, dosed, controlled and administered by Mr Gattefossé. The study of the physiological action, the most suitable carriers, their forms and preparations constitutes an "Aromatherapy", a wide range of efficacious medicines, usually easy to absorb.

The chemical industry as a whole is making progress and undergoing a complete transformation. Aniline dyes may very soon produce asphyxiating gases. Aromatic substances can combat narcosis, accidents, fainting and bacteria. The most learned scientists do not eschew their study and use them. What discoveries have been made and how much has yet to be revealed!

Dr FOVEAU DE COURMELLES

FOREWORD

With thirty years of experimentation behind us, we can now "take stock" and assess the situation. The numerous papers, theses and observations made on this subject by the large number of scientists interested since 1907, when our work on the subject commenced, and published in journals and special bulletins, are hard and sometimes impossible to find. We summarize the bulk of them here and give our readers the names of reference works.

Browsing through these pages, doctors and chemists will be surprised at the large number of aromatic substances which can be used in medicine and the wide variety of their chemical functions. However, two properties are common to them all: they are *Volatile* and they are *Aromatic*.

Extracted, for the most part, from aromatic plants, they constitute the culmination of certain of the benefits provided by these plants, to which the ancients attributed rare properties.

Essential oils have been analysed, their constituents isolated and then reproduced synthetically; there is no appreciable difference between a pure constituent obtained by analysis and the same constituent reproduced synthetically other than, at times, a change in the nature of imperceptible impurities which can taint them and slightly alter their properties.[2]

Incidentally, all plants have a smell, and consequently contain a volatile oil:[3] essential oils not yet extracted will be put to good use in the fullness of time.

However, the most important – and also the most surprising – factor to bear in mind is this: the whole natural world is scented, yet until today no one has sought to know why. Man, animals, plants, even minerals at times, give off a smell. And we even have a sense to distinguish good smells from bad ones. The former please us, the latter repel or revolt us. Is this not because the former can be beneficial to us and the latter harmful?

All peoples with only a rudimentary hygiene use aromatic plants for prophylactic and therapeutic purposes. Will the civilised world ever make the effort to discover why there are good and bad smells? Will science one day tell us the reason for their life-enhancing action or, alternatively, the dangers they harbour?[4]

Do aromatic plants contain substances of value to man? Do their volatile principles have greater curative powers than their fixed extracts? Do the aromatic substances in any way modify the action of the non-aromatic, make them less toxic or widen their field of application?

Are aromatic substances similar to vitamins?[5] Is not their role in the plant world the same as that of hormones in the animal kingdom? Are they not consequently indispensable to plant life and valuable to human life?[6]

So many pressing questions – but we will answer them as best we can on the basis of our experience, meagre as it is before the immensity of the problem.

At least the questions have been raised. We have begun to decipher this immense, as yet uncharted domain. Besides their antiseptic and bactericidal properties widely used today (in part thanks to our work), essential oils possess anti-toxic and antiviral properties, have a powerful vitalizing action, an undeniable healing power and extensive therapeutic properties, as we have demonstrated and this work documents. A number of patent medicines already exploit these properties and human lives have been saved by their use. But the future has a far greater role in store for them.

Today, essential oils gratify our sense of smell. We use them "for pleasure" and, unwittingly, for our health. We now need to learn to understand them better and make better use of them. Many researchers, armed with the information we have provided, are forging ahead. The momentum is there. This is why we are happy to popularise our initial discoveries in this avenue which holds the prospect of many new applications. We have no illusions, however, about the level of perfection of our first steps. We and our colleagues have been exploring an almost entirely unknown terrain. We may make errors and omissions – but this is only natural: today's truth is but the embryo of tomorrow's.

But we must start somewhere.

This is what we offer our readers.

Réné-Maurice GATTEFOSSÉ
1936

chapter one

HUMAN, ANIMAL AND PLANT SMELLS

If man knew, if he had not lost
his primordial wisdom, he would find
that he has not been expelled from Eden.
He still lives in Paradise, but he does not
know it because the knowledge has been
expelled from his spirit.

Eleanor Sinclair Rohde
(The Old English Herbals)

HUMAN SMELLS

Humans undoubtedly have smells which, although barely perceptible outdoors or from one individual, become quite distinct in a closed environment or in a crowd. When you enter a
dormitory, a bedroom, a living room or a theatre or if you have
simply breathed fresh morning air outside and then return to the
closed room where you slept, you perceive the smells of man
immediately – and by no means always with pleasure.

Travellers and explorers have all noticed that every race seems to
have and emanate a particular scent, a unique smell. An oriental or
black person does not have the same smell as a white person. People
of the same race, the same tribe, do not notice their own smell
because they are accustomed to it, but they certainly notice the
smells of foreigners. The Spanish conquistadors said that the natives
they used as trackers never failed when it came to identifying
someone of their own race, a white or a black. During the war of
1914, French soldiers occupying a building, an underground pas-
sage or a trench easily detected the nationality of the previous
occupants, whether Belgian, English or German, by sniffing the air.
The quarters of black troops smelt completely different from those
of Asians.

Claudius Roux who studied this question in depth in his work
entitled *Produits odorants d'origine animale* [Aromatic substances
of animal origin] which has been a great source of information for
this work, adds that in all races, a woman's body is, if not more
aromatic, at least more fragrant than a man's, without, of course,
any use of floral perfume or other substance made by a perfumer.

This smell, particular to women, has been noticed throughout
the ages, this "odor di femina", as the Italians say, a smell which
varies from woman to woman and which is more noticeable during
their menstrual periods, to the extent that some women cannot be in
the company of other people without immediately attracting attention, even after taking all possible hygienic precautions.

In his book *Le Parfum de la Femme* [The Scent of Woman],
Galopin noted the natural odour of musk and amber some women
have, able to scent a whole bath. Ash blonds, he adds, smell more
particularly of amber. Redheads apparently have a less pleasant
smell.

History reminds us that Madame de Maintenon smelt of musk
whereas Agnès Sorel smelt of violets and Diane de Poitiers of amber.

It is claimed that in Japan, the smells of marriageable young people are taken into consideration. The military service entrance examination also takes them into account.

There is a category of human smells which stands in contrast to the stench of decay: a decomposing corpse gives off fetid odours. However, some corpses not only do not decompose but, instead, mummify, and also give off a pleasant scent. Hagiographical works often speak of such fragrant smells coming from saints' bodies; it is the smell of sanctity, in its true sense; however, it is not limited to the religious. It has also been witnessed fairly often in normal mortals. Perhaps this smell is due to total chastity and a severely restricted diet.

Dr Paoli, an Italian doctor, wrote about one of his patients whose body showed no sign of decomposing twenty days after his death but instead gave off a pleasant scent.

It is said of Saint Lydwine of Schiedam in Holland (1380–1433), whose life was a continual martyrdom because of the disabilities which plagued her until her demise, that in the cell in which her suffering confined her to her bed, the air was delicately fragrant. This saint lived in a near permanent state of ecstasy which apparently had an effect on the smell of her human secretions.

It is also said (Professor Ferrua) that in convents, the sweet-smelling hormones emanating during the state of ecstasy make such a state in some way contagious. The same author adds that theologians have cited the exhalation of perfumes from the body as a phenomenon common to a number of saints. Saint Dominique's hands gave off a subtle odour. Saint Francis of Sales' body gave off a less agreeable smell when he chastised himself or after fasting for a prolonged period. All of these facts undeniably attest to a secretory disorder in the sweat glands caused by the stimulation of the nervous system.

While it has been noted that human smells are strongest during sexual arousal, it is not true to say that this is the only time that fragrant hormones are released. They are affected by state of mind, emotions and voluntary actions (*Le parfum de la femme et le sens olfactif dans l'amour*) [The perfume of woman and the olfactory sense in love], A. Galopin, 1886). Thus, they are not specifically sexual secretions, but a more generalized exudation from a number of glands.

ANIMAL SMELLS

Smells sometimes emanate from the whole body of an animal, especially in the male. This is true, for example, of wild animals and billy-goats. These smells attract and excite the female. They are much fainter or totally absent in castrated males. In female animals, the sexual odour is more localized around the sexual organs. In both sexes, the odours are stronger during the mating season.

Many animals have special scent glands, the organs producing odorous substances. The most well-known secretions from these glands are those produced by the beaver, the civet and the musk deer.

However, all animals, even lower organisms, have smells which are perceptible to a greater or lesser degree. Molluscs give off a strong scent. This is particularly true of the musk octopus which, according to Pliny, was dried and reduced to powder for use as a perfume. These molluscs, in fact, constitute the basic diet of the sperm whale and can be considered as one of the ingredients which produce ambergris.

Onyx, used in ancient times in the preparation of sanctuary incense, was extracted from certain large gastropod molluscs such as the *Strombus* and the *Murex*, the opercula of which were so named because of their resemblance to a claw.

However, the most varied odorous species are found in the vast world of insects.

In *Formicidae*, according to Ettimiles, the nympha emit a strong scent of nutmeg; lice are known for their fetid smell; the musk beetle, the tiger beetle, *Brachinus* or bombardier beetles, ladybirds and many other insects give off their own particular smells.

H. Fabre, the entomologist, carefully studied olfaction in insects and concluded that scented secretions were important in reproduction and therefore useful for the preservation of the species.

Professor Raphaël Dubois, who studied not only insects' odours but also scent-emitting organs, also came to this conclusion. Raphaël Dubois notes, for example, that in African *Mylothris* and *Teracolus* (one variety of which has a smell similar to syringa and another similar to jasmine), only the males are scented on the upper side of the wings. The aromatic substance is produced by the glands located at the base of their feather-shaped scales.[7]

P. A. Dixey claims that scents are emitted by an animal at will when, as the British author prudishly says, "it wants to start a family"; the more specific the insect's intentions, the stronger the scent.

In other butterflies, both sexes give off a – sometimes unpleasant – scent, but it does seem to be a defense mechanism against insectivorous birds.

This question of the sense of smell in insects has, in the past, fuelled controversy with regard to ants among some eminent scientists, such as Balbiani, Braber, Lehmann, Lubbock, Perris, Plateau, Forel and Gantschi of Kairouan.

There are many aromagenic mammals.

In his *Principes d'adénisation* [Principles of adenine production] (1859), Cornay attempted to distinguish between truly scented mammals, such as the musk deer, and mammals which produce odorous substances or which have glands which produce odorous substances. This distinction does not appear to be well founded and has not been adopted.

Odorous mammals are divided into seven groups or orders: marsupials, rodents, ruminants, pachyderms, cetaceans, carnivores and insectivores.

In these seven groups, 24 families with 40 species are clearly aromagenic (Claudius Roux, op. cit.).

There is no point in listing them all here; however, we should mention those from which fragrant secretions are obtained either for use as medicines and perfumes, such as castoreum, musk and amber, or as perfumes and aphrodisiacs, such as civet.[8]

Many studies have been conducted on the beaver. In ancient times, the beaver was the hero of legends; the most famous legend has it that, when the beaver is pursued by hunters, he bites off his scented testicles and leaves them as a ransom for his life. Needless to say, the testicles are not the scent glands and, furthermore, since these glands and the testicles are found inside the body, the beaver could not possibly bite them off. On either side of the cloaca into which the genital and urinary systems open, according to Chatin and Raillet, there are two pairs of secretory glands. The bottom ones produce a liquid of the consistency of honey, which thickens with age and makes the animal's fur waterproof. The elongated upper glands secrete *castoreum verum*, are 8 to 13 centimetres long and open either into the vagina or the preputial canal. Castoreum is dried and often cured, to preserve it, before it is sold. Its aroma is thus difficult to detect at first but its infusion in alcohol has a pleasant, persistent odour, reminiscent of musk and with similar effects.

Under its abdomen between the navel and the penis, the musk deer has an internal rounded pouch, six to seven centimetres long and three to five centimetres wide, opening close to the preputial aperture.

The mucous membrane in this pouch has many folds; follicles located in them secrete musk.

Dry musk comes in the form of a blackish granular substance with a strong distinctive odour which is pleasant when diluted.

The sperm whale does not produce ambergris from a special gland. It seems to be the product of an accumulation of odorous substances from the octopus which form a semi-pasty bezoar which hardens when dried.

Although ambergris cannot be compared to castoreum or musk, its physiological properties seem to be fairly similar.

Brandes' analysis indicates that castoreum contains cholesterol, fat, a volatile oil and water-soluble matter.

According to Guibourt and Planchon, and Geiger and Reimann, musk also contains cholesterol, fats, a bitter resin, water-soluble salts and a volatile substance analysed by Ruszika.

Galen recommends castoreum in these terms: "It is a well-known medicine with great and varied properties". *Le Grand Herbier en François* [The Great French Herbal] (1548) cites it as an aphrodisiac. Pierre d'Apono in his *Conciliator* (quoted by Cabanès) advises old men on their death beds that they can prolong their existence by inhaling saffron and castoreum mixed with wine. In his *Dioscorides*, Mattioli quotes Pliny, saying that castoreum is good for people with falling disease (epilepsy), it cures toothache and can be used as an antidote to poison.

According to Olaüs Magnus, castoreum is the best specific for the plague and is effective for all diseases.

Castoreum was still highly regarded in the 17th and 18th centuries. Jean Marie Mayer, a doctor in Ulm, Jean Frank in 1685, and then Lémery all recommend it as "alleviating viscous humours, fortifying the brain, stimulating menstruation in a woman, resistant to putrefaction, and eliminating bad humours through perspiration. It can be used in cases of epilepsy, paralysis and apoplexy". The recent work by Chevallier and Baudrimont on Falsifications lists castoreum as an antispasmodic and antihysteric in the form of pills, enemas and potions.

In the article entitled "Tincture of Castor", the British Pharmaceutical Codex says that castoreum has a definite action on the heart, that it improves blood circulation and strengthens peripheral vessels.

Musk is even better. It fortifies and is a tonic for heart irregularities, coldness and palpitations. It fortifies the brain and heals deep-rooted headaches "caused by an excess of phlegmatic humour". It is an aphrodisiac, according to Mattioli and Lémery. It fortifies the heart and the brain, stimulates semen and eliminates wind. It is also applied to the womb to combat vapours. Chevallier and Baudrimont say that it is a powerful stimulant used to treat nervous illnesses, typhoid fever, tetanus, convulsions, whooping cough and hysteria. An abundant body of literature cited by Claudius Roux praises the incomparable merits of musk.

Ambergris and civet have similar properties. Animal perfumes are without dispute effective at very low doses. In Germany, doctors protested when it was rumoured that these substances were to be removed from the Codex.

In treating any disease which causes general depression, it is perhaps wrong to disregard these powerful substances which stimulate bodily functions while calming the nervous system.

Recently, surprising successes have been reported in cases of delirium tremens, convulsive ailments, stridulous laryngitis, typhoid fever and even in one case of rheumatic fever.

Would you not say that the aromatic principles secreted by animals, although specifically sexual hormones, have, as might be expected, a considerable effect on the whole physical system of an animal?

Hormones are catalysts of vital functions, with a mechanism we still do not fully understand. They are also naturally highly concentrated and keep well.

We cannot deny that while odorous secretions from man and animals are related to certain psychological influences (female civets are led past the cages of male civets to increase their production of perfume), they are also related to certain biological and pathological states. Doctors and surgeons can recognize the specific odours of certain diseases and can tell from the smell how the disease is progressing and when the patient is beginning to recover.

Pathological odours are so characteristic that M. Roussy was led to assert that diseases are due to the presence of odorous volatile elements. It is more likely that toxins have an unpleasant smell whereas antitoxins have a pleasant one. Thus the role of the sense of smell could be explained as that of sensing danger or inducing one to stay in fragrant and healthy environments in the interest of preserving the species. Do plant essences play the role of substitute antitoxins?

We can state that humans are malodorous when ill, yet smell pleasant to varying degrees when recovering and in full health, have a stronger smell during sexual arousal and an intense and characteristic smell in states of psychic exaltation such as ecstasy.

We have seen that a corpse smells pleasant when undergoing a natural preservation process and in the absence of any phenomenon of decay.

Upon reflection, there are some disturbing yet clear facts in this area of study which may point to a whole therapeutic concept based on odours.

PLANT SMELLS

It has been said that all plants have a smell: every plant has a scent to a sensitive nose.[9] The sense of smell plays a major role in diet. All animals and people smell whatever they are about to eat or drink. It is usually the nose which indicates whether a dish is fresh and safe to eat. Of course, the nose is not infallible and there are plenty of substances which smell good but are dangerous. Nonetheless, it would be foolish to deny that the sense of smell, like the other senses, contributes to the preservation of the individual as well as the species. By studying the issue in this light, we can understand the importance of fragrances, whatever their source.

Aromatic plants are those which contain enough essential oil to give an excess of aromatic essence when distilled by steam;[10] this essence separates from the condensed water because its density differs from that of water. However, all plants produce fragrant water when processed in a still. This water contains a certain amount of essence but it is diffuse or dissolved to such an extent that it is generally not considered worthwhile collecting it.

Distilled water from plants contains up to 0.20 grams of odorous substances per litre and sometimes more when the constituents are highly water-soluble. Rosewater, for example, can contain 50 to 60 centigrams of phenylethyl alcohol.

Essences can be extracted from distilled water by adding ether, which attaches to the oils.

The plant concerned can also be processed with sulphuric ether or with petroleum ether. This produces a mixture of essential oil and ethereal extract which is rinsed with alcohol. Only the volatile parts dissolve in ethanol and they are separated in this way from the other soluble substances in the ether. These are known as "volatile-solvent essences"[11] in contrast to "steam-distilled" essences.

All the experiments mentioned are conducted using entirely volatile essential oils and no unpurified oleoresinous essences extracted with petroleum ether. The properties of the non-volatile substances found with these essences are radically different and they are sometimes highly toxic. This distinction is of the utmost importance.

Some essential oils, such as those from lemon, orange, bergamot and citron peel etc., are obtained by expression, without distillation. They therefore contain a fixed, non-volatile residue which does not dissolve in alcohol. This residue does not have the properties of the volatile substances and these essences need to be distilled before being used for medicinal purposes.[12]

Numerous scientists have studied the formation of essences in plants, including: Bouchardat, Grimaux, Gerber, Charabot, Moureu, Dupont, Tardy, Barbier, Haller, Naudin, Hébert, Laloue, Ripert, Miss Popovici, Francesconi, Tschirich, Moreau, Guilliermond and Mangenot, to name but a few. The general, if not unanimous, opinion is that essential oils are created in a plant's chlorophyllous organs.

Just before the first inflorescence appears, as Charabot reports, the essence is rich in terpenic (non-oxidized) hydrocarbons in particular and accumulates in the green parts of the plant.

At a further stage in flowering, when the flower has fulfilled some of its functions, the quantity of essence in the green parts of the plant decreases while it increases in the flowers.

When the seed matures, transportation from the leaf to the stem and the flower ceases, the amount of volatile oil in the flowers decreases but increases once again in the chlorophyllous organs, unless the plant, having completed its annual cycle, withers completely. During these stages, the terpenic compounds oxidize into alcohols and then etherify or convert into aldehydes or ketones, particularly where respiration is greatest (A. Dubosq).

This is why, for example, oil of turpentine from the pinaster is composed almost entirely of pinene and resin in the trunk, from which it is extracted by tapping. In the leaves, however, the essence contains terpene alcohols, terpineol, borneol and bornyl ethers, as well as residual terpenes from a local function not yet determined.

It is thus apparent that chemical phenomena which modify the composition of a plant's aromatic substances are closely linked to the plant's physiological functions. Experience has shown that factors which intensify the chlorophyllous function also promote the etherification of terpene in alcohols.

This is therefore a biological process very similar to hormonal processes in animals. Essences are thus extremely powerful and their effects are manifold.

The effect of light is quite considerable. When aromatic plants are placed in darkness, the odorous compounds are destroyed so that they can either help to form tissue or provide energy which the plant lacks in the absence of light. Terpenes are therefore the first stage in the formation of the aromatic substance, whereas oxygenated substances are the most developed, and are involved in the plant's reproductive and vital functions and the formation of seed or reproductive organs.

In short, essential oils play the same role in plants as hormones play in animals.[13] It is a sexual role, that of preservation of the species, of tissue formation and of the triggering of other functions. Essential oils probably also play a defensive role by accumulating vital energy. Today, as in ancient times, volatile ingredients can be said to be "vital ingredients".

The following chapters will show whether the term "plant hormones", used by Professor Ferrua, is an exaggeration.

As for minerals, many of them give off an odour either in their normal state or when they are rubbed or heated. The smell of tin when it is bent is well known. Antimony and iodine also have individual smells, but the barely perceptible odours of some minerals have not always been noted with the interest they merit. A study of these smells could perhaps teach us even more about the mechanism of sense of smell and about the nature of smells themselves.

chapter two

THE CLASSIFICATION OF ESSENTIAL OILS

E ssential oils contain constituents which possess almost the full range of chemical functions. The simplest are hydrocarbons, constituting the terpene family, of the type p-cymene, $C^{10}H^{14}$, which is similar to pinene, a constituent of oil of turpentine. The other constituents can almost all be classified as various stages in terpene development:

alcohols, characterised by the OH group;
aldehydes, characterised by the CHO group;
ketones, characterised by the CO group;
acids, characterised by the COOH group;
and esters which are compounds of acids with alcohols.

In addition to these constituents, which make up the main part of essential oils, many other substances are found, which we will discuss later, and which account for only a small part of each essential oil.

Charabot and Dupont attempted to establish a rational classification system for essential oils based on the qualitative dominance of one of the above-mentioned constituents in each essential oil.

The first family includes those essences having, as their principal constituent, a terpene alcohol or ethers of this alcohol, for instance: geranium oil, which contains the alcohols geraniol and citronellol and their ethers; and bergamot, lavender, neroli and ylang-ylang essences, which contain mainly linalol and linalyl ethers; etc.

The second family includes essences which contain mainly aldehydes, such as bitter almond essence (benzaldehyde) and the essences of cinnamon bark (cinnamic aldehyde), lemon and lemongrass (citral) etc.

Ketones characterise the third family: iris (irone), wormwood (thujone) and caraway (carvone).

The fourth comprises lactones.

The fifth family includes phenol essences: clove and cinnamon leaf (eugenol), thyme, wild thyme (thymol and carvacrol) and anise (anethol).

The sixth family comprises aldehyde and phenol essences.

The seventh, oxide essences (eucalyptus, niaouli).

The eighth, essences with a terpene or sesquiterpene as their main constituent.

The ninth family comprises essential oils which have a fatty alcohol ether as their main constituent; and the tenth, sulphuric compound oils (garlic, mustard etc.).

A provisional eleventh family comprises essences with unknown constituents.

The potential medical applications of the various essential oils should be indicated by their classification but, unfortunately, the matter is not so simple as essences contain substances which, although not dominant in terms of quantity, do influence potential applications by their presence alone.

If we take a look at the first family, for example, we immediately note that bergamot essence and lavender essence are placed side by side as containing mainly linalyl acetate. Yet terpenes comprise over half the weight of the first and only 10 to 15% of the second. As we will see later, the presence of this proportion of terpene substantially modifies the qualities of essential oils, particularly with regard to their medicinal applications.

In the second family, lemongrass essence, with a 75% citral content, is found together with lemon essence, which contains only 4%. The first contains 15 to 20% methylheptenone and the second, 90% limonene.

Java citronella essence, which contains almost as much aldehyde (citronellal) as it does alcohol (geraniol), could just as well be placed in the first category of essences as in the second, whereas Ceylon citronella oil contains only alcohols and no aldehyde.

With phenols, a distinction should be made between those which are slightly caustic (eugenol, thymol, carvacrol) and those which are not at all caustic (anethole, estragole).

This is why Charabot and Dupont's initial classification needs to be replaced, as far as medicinal applications are concerned, by another, in which only the non-terpene content is taken into account, for we will see that all terpenes have special and almost constant properties which mask or denature the properties of the other constituents. It is always preferable (and this can be easily demonstrated) to use terpeneless essences.[14] This is why we have devised a new classification of essential oils "after terpene removal".

THE CLASSIFICATION OF TERPENELESS ESSENCES

If we consider essences with their terpenes removed, we immediately see that the disadvantages of Charabot and Dupont's initial classification disappear. To take our previous examples, terpeneless bergamot essence, consisting mainly of linalyl acetate takes its natural place alongside terpeneless lavender, which has a very similar composition. Without terpenes, lemon and lemongrass essences are closely allied, both being composed principally of citral.

Clove oil without caryophyllene is almost pure eugenol, and terpeneless thyme essences contain, almost exclusively, phenols (thymol and carvacrol).[15] Terpeneless mint essences contain primarily menthol and no menthone (a potentially dangerous ketone). In this new classification, therefore, substances which act in a similar way and which are interchangeable are grouped together.

Moreover, the removal of terpenes eliminates the previously mentioned non-volatile impurities found in essences obtained by extraction or expression.

The following is a brief classification of terpeneless essences:

First family: essences with terpene alcohols and their ethers as their main constituents.
Second family: aldehydes.
Third family: ketones.
Fourth family: lactones.
Fifth family: phenols.
Seventh family: oxides (oxide ethers).
Eighth family: terpenes.

We will not include natural essential oils in the eighth family (terpenes), as no essential oil is simply a pure terpene, with the possible exception of oil of turpentine, but rather all the terpenes extracted from the above essential oils.

We find that the essences of lime, caraway and orange, the main constituent of which, in terms of quantity, is a terpene, can be put in the second (aldehydes) or the third family (ketones) respectively because the constituent which is actually of interest is the least important in terms of quantity.

This approach of no longer classifying natural compounds but rather pure, isolated constituents also leads us to a new classification – that of the pure constituents.

CLASSIFICATION OF AROMATIC CONSTITUENTS

First family: alcohols.
   First sub-family: ethers – salts.
Second family: aldehydes.
Third family: ketones.

Fourth family: lactones.
Fifth family: phenols.
Eighth family: terpenes, sesquiterpenes.

Essential oils also contain many other substances which can be isolated in their pure state. A number of these substances will probably be found to have valuable properties. We are still at a more general stage, but once the main properties of the most plentiful substances are recognised, it will be possible to concentrate on the study of the rarer constituents.

Moreover, the chemical industry is creating, from the individual constituents, substances which do not exist in nature, or which are too costly if taken from their natural origins. These aromatic substances, or Synthetic Fragrances, also have the properties of natural aromatic substances and their study will be extremely rewarding.

CHARACTERISTICS OF SOME AROMATIC SUBSTANCES

It is important to show that terpeneless essences are natural "compounds" quite distinct from their main constituent which is often believed to be the main agent of the results obtained.

The following table gives the two principal constants (density and optical rotation) of essential oils, the corresponding terpeneless essences, terpenes (non-oxidised hydrocarbons) eliminated during the process of terpene removal and, if applicable, the main constituent.

NAME OF ESSENCE	DENSITY	OPTICAL ROTATION
Angelica, essential oil	0.8935	+ 15°12
Angelica, terpeneless essence	0.9154	− 3°48
Bay, essential oil	0.980	− 3°
Bay, terpeneless essence	1.027	− 0°98
Bay, terpenes	0.8063	− 6°50
Methyl chavicol	0.9850	0°

NAME OF ESSENCE	DENSITY	OPTICAL ROTATION	
Bergamot, essential oil	0.8828	+	7°10
Bergamot, terpeneless essence	0.8848	−	8°81
Bergamot, terpenes	0.8482	+	63°16
Linalyl acetate	0.9130	+	6°
Bitter orange, essential oil	0.8593	+	58°87
Bitter orange, terpeneless	0.9106	+	6°29
Bitter orange, terpenes	0.8449	+	75°
Limonene	0.8470	+	105°
Caraway, essential oil	0.911	+	80°
Caraway, terpeneless essence	0.9634	+	58°2
Caraway, terpenes	0.849	+	105°5
Carvone	0.964	+	59°
Limonene	0.847	+	105°
Cardamom, essential oil	0.9364	+	30°72
Cardamom, terpeneless essence	0.9548	+	45°93
Cardamom, terpenes	0.8626	−	8°30
Celery, essential oil	0.8614	+	92°4
Celery, terpeneless essence	0.930	+	27°5
Celery, terpenes	0.8477	+	108°6
Limonene	0.847	+	105°
Cinnamon bark, essential oil	1.020	−	1°
Cinnamon bark, terpeneless ess.	1.032	−	0°32
Cinnamic aldehyde	1.054		0°
Cinnamon leaf, essential oil	1.0544	+	0°14
Cinnamon leaf, terpeneless ess.	1.0583	−	0°52
Eugenol	1.0700		0°
Ceylon citronella, essential oil	0.9049	−	10°
Ceylon citronella, terpeneless ess.	0.9139	−	5°
Ceylon citronella, terpenes	0.8383	−	43°
Geraniol	0.880		0°
Coriander, essential oil	0.880	+	10°

NAME OF ESSENCE	DENSITY	OPTICAL ROTATION	
Coriander, terpeneless essence	0.8843	+	8°95
Coriander, terpenes	0.854		
Cubeb, essential oil	0.938	−	10°
Cubeb, terpeneless essence	0.9428	−	10°05
Cubeb, terpenes	0.8662	−	15°45
Calamus, essential oil	0.958	+	9°
Calamus, terpeneless essence	0.910		
Eucalyptus, essential oil	0.912	−	4°50
Eucalyptus, terpeneless essence	0.9382	−	1°72
Eucalyptus, terpenes	0.8677	−	13°
Cineol or eucalyptol	0.930		0°
Fennel, essential oil	0.968	+	8°70
Fennel, terpeneless essence	0.981	+	13°
Fennel, terpenes	0.852	+	37°7
Fenchone	0.950	+	70°
French peppermint, essential oil	0.914	−	17°74
French peppermint, terpeneless ess.	0.922	−	20°
French peppermint, terpenes	0.874	−	25°47
Menthol	0.890	−	49°
Galangal, essential oil	0.9175	−	2°60
Galangal, terpeneless essence	0.9259	−	6°37
Galangal, terpenes	0.8675	+	2°78
Geranium, essential oil	0.891	−	11°
Geranium, terpeneless essence	0.897	−	8°54
Citronellol	0.860	−	4°
Ginger, essential oil	0.880	−	40°
Ginger, terpeneless essence	0.9117	−	11°30
Hyssop, essential oil	0.9399	−	18°
Hyssop, terpeneless essence	0.9531	−	19°5

NAME OF ESSENCE	DENSITY	OPTICAL ROTATION
Hyssop, terpenes	0.8633	− 20°
Pinocamphone	0.966	− 13°42
Java citronella, essential oil	0.882	− 3°
Java citronella, terpeneless	0.8897	+ 0°10
Citronellal	0.8538	− 3°
Juniper, essential oil	0.8515	− 8°50
Juniper, terpeneless essence	0.913	
Lavender, essential oil	0.880	− 8°
Lavender, terpeneless essence	0.8967	− 3°6
Lavender, terpenes	0.830	
Linalyl acetate	0.913	+ 6°
Lemon, essential oil	0.854	+ 54°
Lemon, terpeneless essence	0.8966	− 8°53
Citral	0.8955	0°
Limonene	0.847	+ 105°
Lime, essential oil	0.880	+ 32°
Lime, terpeneless essence	0.9165	+ 1°
Mandarin, essential oil	0.8566	+ 71°
Mandarin, terpeneless essence	0.9529	− 0°95
Mandarin, terpenes	0.8476	+ 74°4
Limonene	0.847	+ 105°
Norwegian pine, essential oil	0.8689	+ 5°
Norwegian pine, terpeneless ess.	0.9284	+ 11°64
Pinene	0.864	+ 48°6
Petitgrain, essential oil	0.892	− 1°73
Petitgrain, terpeneless essence	0.8972	− 6°24
Petitgrain, terpenes	0.8278	+ 28°4
Pimenta leaf, essential oil	1.0347	− 6°14
Pimenta leaf, terpeneless essence	1.0623	− 1°

NAME OF ESSENCE	DENSITY	OPTICAL ROTATION
Pimenta leaf, terpenes		− 46°2
Rosemary, essential oil	0.915	+ 5°
Rosemary, terpeneless essence	0.9441	+ 10°
Rosemary, terpenes	0.8568	− 4°
Borneol	1.011	+ 37°
Sage, essential oil	0.9263	+ 11°76
Sage, terpeneless essence	0.9315	+ 11°26
Sage, terpenes	0.8817	+ 3°65
Borneol	1.011	+ 37°
Sassafras, essential oil	1.070	+ 1°30
Sassafras, terpeneless essence	1.088	+ 2°04
Safrole	1.105	0°
Scots pine, essential oil	0.8751	+ 0°14
Scots pine, terpeneless essence	0.9341	− 0°52
Scots pine, terpenes	0.8584	0°
Star anise, essential oil	0.980	
Star anise, terpeneless essence	0.9856	
Star anise, terpenes	0.8495	+ 98°
Anethol	0.9850	+ 9°65
		+ 102°
Sweet orange, essential oil	0.848	
Sweet orange, terpeneless essence	0.894	
Sweet orange, terpenes	0.847	
Limonene	0.847	
Thyme, essential oil	0.900	− 5°
Thyme, terpeneless essence	0.933	− 2°
Thyme, terpenes	0.860	− 13°96
Carvacrol	0.981	
Thymol	0.979	

NAME OF ESSENCE	DENSITY	OPTICAL ROTATION
Wormwood, essential oil	0.9455	+ 27°
Wormwood, terpeneless essence	0.9220	+ 29°4
Wormwood, terpenes	0.8314	− 19°6
Thujone	0.9125	− 10°23

These analyses, the figures of which were obtained by Haensel de Pirna, Jehancard and ourselves, show that terpenes all have one common denominator: they are light. They all weigh in the region of 0.850, whereas terpeneless essences approach or exceed a density of 900 grams per litre.

Terpenes like limonene all differ substantially (usually having a higher value), while terpeneless essences approach optical inactivity, except for essences with a high menthol content.

The pure constituents are rarely identical to the terpeneless essence, which is usually a mixture of various constituents and which, correspondingly, has different properties from those of the pure constituent.

chapter three

ESSENCES IN ANCIENT PHARMACOPOEIAS

All ancient pharmacopoeias are full of information about the use of aromatic plants and it is often difficult to know whether the authors placed more importance on the volatile content than on the whole plant. However, essence of rose is often cited as a constituent in remedies in the Middle Ages and during the Renaissance.[16] The abbess Hildegard recommended lavender water for swollen eyelids and Charlemagne's capitular clergy advocated planting this labiate. In his *Dioscorides*, Mattioli speaks at great length about the properties of plants which produce essences and, M. Chaplet tells us, the formulae of medicines made from rose would fill volumes while we would need an entire library for all the recipes for aromatic remedies.

However, in passing, let us mention a few typical examples. According to Mattioli, the odours of wormwood and anise soothe toothache and earache and reduce fever. "Amber is hot: smelling it fortifies the brain and the heart; it is very good for old people". "Civet placed in the navel is excellent for the womb". "Musk fortifies the heart and is a tonic for all its functions".

According to Dr Blondel (*Les produits odorants du rosier* [The fragrant products of the rosebush]), Athene said that the scent of rose is sought by drinkers to cure the heavy-headed feeling caused by the vapours of wine. Pomet, the seventeenth-century apothecary, also said that the scent of rose is effective in gladdening and fortifying the heart and the stomach. Ambroise Paré maintained that turtles eat savory to heal snake bites; sage, like rosemary, restores vital energy.

It is clear from these examples that therapists believed the odour itself, acting as an aromatic, and not the whole plant, produced the desired effect.

In his *Dictionnaire des drogues simples* [Dictionary of Simple Drugs] (1798), Lémery summarised much of the information from previous ages. Without attaching too great importance to his words, we should nevertheless take note of them. Tradition, the collective memory of empirical knowledge going back to the first civilizations, should not be simply dismissed.

The following are the traditional properties of aromatic plants according to Lémery:

Angelica	Warming, stomachic, sudorific, vulnerary, against the plague, fevers and bites of rabid dogs.

Anise	Warming, stomachic, pectoral, carminative, digestive, galactagogue.
Apium (wild celery)	Pectoral, stimulates the appetite, carminative, vulnerary, hysteric, expectorant.
Asafoetida	Hysteric, sudorific.
Balsam of tolu	Against gangrene, rheumatism, sciatica, asthma, for the nerves.
Basil (C)	Diuretic, emmenagogue, cleansing; against venom, wind, for respiration, the brain, nerves, heart, resolves and aids digestion.
Bdellium[17]	Digestive, sudorific, desiccant, stimulates the appetite, against empyema and venom, for childbirth.
Benzoin	Incisive, penetrating, attenuant; against pulmonary ulcers and gangrene.
Bergamot (Ph)	Warming, cephalic, stomachic.
Cade	Digestive, emollient, resolvent, nervine, vulnerary; against scabies and pains.
Camphor	For hysterical women, respiration, scurvy, gangrene; against venom, the vapours, intermittent fevers.
Canada balsam	Purgative.
Caraway	Incisive, stimulates the appetite, carminative, stomachic, galactagogue; against colics and dizziness.
Chio turpentine and Bijou du Dauphiné	Stimulates the appetite, against stones, renal colics, kidney and bladder ulcers,

	urine retention, gonorrhoea, cleanses and heals wounds; against headaches.
Cinnamon (I)	Emmenagogue, stomachic, warming, against venom and sudorific.
Clary sage	Stimulates the appetite, hysteric, emmenagogue; for childbirth, makes a wine inebriating.
Clove (I)	Warming, cephalic, for the teeth, against catarrh.
Clove-nutmeg or Clove-cinnamon	Cephalic, stomachic, stimulates the appetite, against wind and venom.
Copaiba	Against rheumatism, cleanses and binds wounds.
Coriander	Stomachic, digestive, against wind and bad breath.
Costus (S)	Emmenagogue, for the digestion and kidneys, against fever.
Cumin	Resolvent, digestive, attenuant, carminative, emmenagogue and diuretic.
Dittany of Crete	Stimulates the appetite, digestive, warming, emmenagogue, for childbirth, to remove obstructions, for venom and perspiration.
Galbanum	Emmenagogue, stimulates the functions of the organs and the womb, against venom and the vapours.
Geranium	Cleansing, astringent, vulnerary, dissolves blood clots.

Genepi (Artemisia spicata)	Sudorific, against pleurisy.
Goat's rue	Sudorific, against the plague, epilepsy, snake bites, venom and worms.
Helichrysum	Vermifuge, stimulates the appetite, vulnerary, emmenagogue, dissolves blood clots.
Iris	Incisive, attenuant, penetrating, softens and cleanses.
Jasmine	Stimulates the appetite, emollient, for childbirth, colds and against pleurisy.
Juniper	Sudorific, eliminates bad breath.
Kidney vetch	For sores and wounds, cleanses and fortifies.
Labdanum	To soften, for the digestion, attenuant, resolutive, fortifying, to stop bleeding.
Lavender	For the brain, nerves, apoplexy, paralysis, lethargy, epilepsy, rheumatism, resistant to deterioration, aids perspiration, eliminates wind, emmenagogue.
Lavender Stoechas	Attenuant, cleansing, cephalic, stimulates the appetite, hysteric, for the brain, the urine; against melancholy and venom, emmenagogue.
Lemon	Stomachic, digestive; against venom.
Liquidambar	Softens, matures, resolvent, unites; tonic for the womb, cuts, rheumatism, sciatica and the nerves.

Origanum	Cephalic, stomachic, carminative, hysteric, cleansing, stimulates the appetite, respiratory, asthmatic, against jaundice, for milk and sweat.
Mastic	Astringent, analgesic, tightens the fibres of the stomach, stops vomiting, diarrhoea, fortifies, aids digestion.
Melissa	For the heart, the brain, the stomach, emmenagogue, against apoplexy, epilepsy, dizziness, melancholy, malignant fevers and the plague.
Mint	For the brain, heart and stomach; eliminates wind, stimulates thought and the memory, vermifuge, cleansing, stimulates the appetite, emmenagogue, helps childbirth and respiration.
Opopanax	Softens, attenuates, digests, resists deterioration; against wind and hysteria.
Pennyroyal (T, A)	Stimulates the appetite, attenuant, resolvent, carminative, emmenagogue, cervical, against colic.
Peru balsam	For the heart, brain and stomach, against gangrene, sweating, wounds, cold humours and scurvy.
Pine	Diuretic, against toothache.
Rhodium wood	Warming, cephalic.
Rose	Astringent, cleansing, stomachic; against vomiting, diarrhoea, bleeding.
Rue (T, A)	Incisive, attenuant, discussive, emmenagogue; against the vapours,

colic with flatulence, bites of rabid dogs
and snake bites.

Sage (T, A)	Cephalic, nervine, hysteric, stomachic, resolvent, stimulates the appetite; against paralysis, lethargy, apoplexy, catarrh, stimulates saliva production.
Sassafras (C)	Incisive, penetrating, stimulates the appetite, sudorific, cardiac, for resistance to venom, fortifies the sight and brain; against catarrh and sciatica.
Savin (T, A)	Incisive, attenuant, penetrating, emmenagogue, for childbirth, for cleansing wounds; against scabies and ringworm.
Savory	Stimulates the appetite, penetrating, attenuant, for the stomach, respiration, urine, earache, eliminates humours, fortifies the nerves and sight.
Star anise	Warming, carminative, stomachic.
Styrax	Incisive, attenuant, emollient, very resolvent; for the brain.
Tansy (T, A)	Incisive, penetrating, carminative, hysteric; against renal colics, the vapours and wind.
Thyme (I)	Incisive, penetrating, stimulates the appetite, rarefying; against flatulence and colic, catarrh, asthma, digestive, sudorific, emmenagogue.
Valerian	Cardiac, sudorific, vulnerary, stimulates the appetite, emmenagogue; for the brain, respiration and stomach.

Vanilla	Warming, cephalic, stomachic, carminative, diuretic, stimulates the appetite, attenuates viscous humours, emmenagogue and diuretic.
Verbena	Incisive, attenuant, cephalic, vulnerary, resolvent, stimulates the appetite, galactagogue, against kidney and bladder stones and flatulence with colic.
Wild carrot	Emmenagogue and diuretic, against wind and venom.
Wild thyme (I)	Stimulates the appetite, cephalic, hysteric, emmenagogue; for childbirth, against venom, epilepsy and dizziness; diuretic.
Wormwood (T)	Vermifuge, stimulates the appetite, febrifuge.
Yarrow	Anti-asthmatic.

Editor's Notes on oils
(C) = Carcinogenic (very low-level)
(I) = Irritant
(S) = Sensitiser (possibility of allergic reaction)
(T) = Toxic
(A) = Abortifacient
(Ph) = Photosensitizer (do not expose skin to UV rays after using this oil)

As unsatisfactory as it may be, this list shows us that the properties of essential oils were already well known and that most of the current applications of essential oils were already standard.

The action of fragrances on the sexual organs, the use of certain balms and essences for dressing wounds, their action against venom, snake bites, rabid dog bites and generally all strong toxins, as well as many other applications, are clearly stated in ancient codices.

They can now be selected and studied more methodically and with better equipment than in the past.

We can see quite clearly that modern-day pharmacopoeias make, as Montaigne so aptly says, "less use" of perfumes than they could. Perhaps this century will be remembered for remedying this error.

ESSENCES IN EXOTIC
PHARMACOPOEIAS

Pharmacopoeias themselves were derived from primitive religions. All ancient rites used spices or aromatic plants, burned in their natural state (juniper, rosemary, pine, wormwood) or as drugs (gums, resins, balsams). These methods preceded the use of incense in modern religious services, but their purpose was the same: to create an emotional atmosphere conducive to the manifestation of the divinity or psychic states conducive to prophesying. And last but not least, the atmosphere in temples was healthy from the physiological viewpoint (illnesses of pathogenic origin were eliminated).

Exotic pharmacopoeias are truer to their ancient origins than ours.

It is possible to give only a few examples here. It is evident that all so-called "primitive" peoples and those with a wholly empirical science, which to us appears infantile, prefer aromatic plants as remedies.

Local information is, in any case, invaluable in the study of exotic essential oils and there will doubtless be innumerable occasions where we will be able to prepare efficacious remedies based on indigenous applications.

Many essences are used in Chinese medicine, the worth of which is no longer called into question. One of them, that of *Blumea balsamifera*, is rich in borneol. The Orientals' marked preference for borneol has often been noted, borneol being far superior to camphor for reasons we explain below. All the countries of the Far East import large quantities of crystallised borneol which they use to make highly effective remedies.

Also widely used are essences from the roots of *Paeonia Moutan*, which contains paenol (studied by Nagai, *Berichte* [Reports], 1891); the rhizomes of the *Asarum blumei* Duch (birthworts) which contain safrole; *Juniperus chinensis* essence which contains cedrol and cedrene; that of *Acorus calamus* and ginseng which contains panacene (studied by Oliv. N. Sakai, Tokyo Igakukai, 1917), the vasomotor and narcotic properties of which are well known. The examples we have chosen are essences on which we have scientific documents, but what a wealth of essences have yet to be studied!

From China we also get *Curcuma tinctoria*, the root of which is an aromatic and stimulant; *Crotum tiglium L*, the essence of which is acrid, revulsive and drastic; *Mallotus philippinensis* Mull, taeniafuge;[18] China root, *Smilax China L*, which is a depurative, and many other aromatic drugs, the benefits of which only became apparent to us much later. They also contain very special essences, for example the bark of the *Phellodendron chinense* Schneid. and the *P. Sacchalinense* Sarg., the fruit of the *Euscaphis japonica*, the bark of the *Magnolia denudata* (variety of *Purpurascens* Rehd. and Wils) and of the *Eucommia ulmoides* Oli etc.

Ginseng (*Panax ginseng* Ness.) is a tonic, a stimulant and an aphrodisiac which restores strength to convalescents and women weakened by childbirth. In Indochina, *Tam-Thât* (*Panax repens*) is used instead. It is an araliaceous plant grown by local people and its rhizomes contain a remedy which is much appreciated, particularly in the Yünnan.

According to Valmot de Bomare, the Chinese eagerly traded bales of tea for bales of sage from which they made a medicinal infusion.

In Central Asia (Afghanistan, Turkestan, Northern Judea), where asafoetida is gathered from the roots of various ferula plants (*Umbelliferae, Ferula alliacea*), this root is thought to have digestive, tonic and aphrodisiac qualities. It is used to treat flatulence and all nervous problems of the heart, the respiratory system, the uterus and the ovaries. Asafoetida works through the visceral plexus (Professor Ferrua). Serious cases of hysterical convulsions can be greatly helped by inhalation of the essential oil, stopping attacks almost immediately. It acts on the nervous system more quickly in this way than by oral administration.[19]

Primitive Malays used benzoin in the form of ointments and fumigations for medicinal as well as ceremonial purposes. It was they who taught the natives of Laos how to use and apply this resin.

Essence of Kayaputi, or cajeput, is used in popular medicine on the islands of the Indian Ocean, in China and on all the islands of the Pacific as an antineuralgic, anticholeraic and antihysteric. In the Far East, essences of *Laurus camphora* are most widely used for therapeutic purposes.

Among the Berbers in Africa, we know of the Ser'hin or Sarhina which the Arabs called "Bokhour el berber", the perfume of the Berbers. This aromatic which the Berbers call "Tasserr'int" in their language (which Dr Leared wrote as "Tausserghimt" in the Pharmaceutical Journal, 1873) has manifold beneficial properties; it promotes weight gain, is tonic and useful against stomach pains.

The Tikentest, the Akerkarhà of Arab doctors in the Middle

Ages, is known in Europe under the name of African pellitory and is primarily used as a toothpaste. However, it also gained its reputation by improving fertility in women and by countless other properties bordering on the magic. The use of these two products, Tausserghimt and Tikentest, goes back to ancient times, probably before the time of Moses. They were the basis of a lucrative trade throughout Africa and the Middle East.

Tradition is quite categorical about the benefits of aromatic substances and one need only consult local folklore to gain some insight into the enormous importance attributed to them, both as medicines and as perfumes. The discovery of their properties is often attributed to animals: it is said that the snake rubs itself with anise in the spring because its sight deteriorates over the winter (Perron, *Médecine du Prophète* [The Prophet's Medicine]) and thus distilled anise water is used to treat eye diseases.

Popowia capea is an *Anonaceæ* used in baths in the Ivory Coast, and thought to have tremendous curative properties.

In Madagascar, Dr Charles Ranaïvo, of the Faculty of Medicine of Paris, studied Rambiazana, a helichrysum-type composite, which smells strongly of roses and provides an essential oil we have analysed. Rambiazana has long been used by the Malagasy as an analgesic, antiseptic and disinfectant. It is used to treat pains and rheumatism, dysmenorrhoea and uterine, renal and hepatic colic. It is used internally and externally for all types of sores, for diarrhoea and all mouth diseases, especially ulcerous gingivitis. Rambiazana is carminative and stomachic. It also soothes headaches and aids sleep. Dr Ranaïvo describes a curious use similar to that of other volatile narcotic substances: the aromatic leaves are used to make mangos ripen more rapidly so they can be sold as early fruits.

Other aromatic plants are used in Madagascar and would reward further study. M. Ledreu describes the following: Valuvy root, used to treat gonorrhoea; Ramangoaka root, to treat dysentery; Zana bark to treat vomiting; Dendemo leaves to treat leprosy; Voaseya leaves, used to strengthen sickly children; Voanana leaves to treat colic; Tsianiamposa wood to treat leprosy sores and Tsiborata roots to treat dysentery.

Achillea fragrantissima Forsk, or Quai Sun as the Syrians call it, is used as a tonic. From time immemorial, Chios mastic, or lentisk resin, has been used in the Orient to treat stomach problems, to stop heavy bleeding, to detoxify and to strengthen the gums. Ladanum or labdanum of Cyprus is soporific and resolvent.

Brazilians use copaiba balsam to prevent "diàs" headaches, a type of tetanus which affects newborn infants. This balsam is also used for cystitis, gonorrhoea, colds and bronchitis.

In Australia, Tea tree (*Melaleuca alternifolia*) essence is used to prevent pus forming, to treat boils, carbuncles and skin diseases, particularly tropical impetigo which is so unpleasant, as well as catarrh and other respiratory infections.

We will not dwell on exotic pharmacopoeias any further. Explorers and colonial doctors could add to this list ad infinitum.

One fact remains: from time immemorial, in every country, aromatic plants have always been considered the most effective treatment for the diseases afflicting mankind. In many cases, the essential oil is used, which is evidence that the volatile part is the most effective. This is not because, as some believe, the smell attracts the attention of the uninitiated better and stimulates auto-suggestion in the patient, but rather because volatile aromatic substances have true therapeutic value.

Empiricism has never intentionally erred, for the very basis of its knowledge is experience frequently repeated over a long period of time. Volatile essences have healed people since the dawn of time and we must try to discover why and how.

Essences in Modern Pharmacopoeias

Modern pharmacopoeias do not appear to be making significant progress in the use of volatile essences. Mention of essential oils by recent authors and even information in the Codex seems to be more or less copied from the information of previous centuries.*

We would have hoped for a more thorough documentation in works on medical substances. The following is a summary of what can be found on essences in the *Traité* by Dr Reutter, of the University of Geneva:

Ajowan: (T)	carminative.
Angelica:	local, carminative and stomachic.

---

* *Le Précis de Matière médicale* [Précis of Medical Material] by Planchon et Manceau, 4th édition, contains a wealth of useful information about the therapeutic uses of essential oils; we congratulate the authors on being the first to take this step.

Anise:	carminative, stomachic, emmenagogue, galactogenic, slows the heart rate, increases leucocyte (white blood cells) count and the secretion of milk, saliva and bile.
Atlas cedar:	anti-gonorrhoeic and specific for tuberculosis.
Bergamot: (Ph)	used rarely as stomachic stimulant.
Boldo: (T)	stomach tonic.
Borneo camphor (borneol):	not to be prescribed!!
Cajeput:	antispasmodic, stomachic, diaphoretic, antirheumatic externally.
Celery (wild celery):	in popular medicine, stomachic and diuretic.
Ceylon cinnamon:	antiseptic, stomachic.
Chinese cinnamon:	same use as Ceylon cinnamon.
Clove: (I)	carminative.
Copaiba (balsam):	anti-gonorrhoeic, antiseptic, disinfectant, against catarrh of the bladder and lungs.
Coriander:	stimulant, carminative.
Cypress:	not medicinal.
Dill:	galactagogue, carminative (according to Dioscorides), sudorific and sedative (Middle Ages).

Eucalyptus:	expectorant, stomachic, haemostatic, intestinal astringent.
Fennel:	stomach stimulant, carminative.
Galangal:	disinfectant, antiseptic.
Geranium:	not medicinal.
Japanese camphor:	antispasmodic, cardiac stimulant, antiseptic, sedative for hysteria and nocturnal erections, bronchial catarrh, odontalgic.
Juniper:	prescribed as a substitute for oil of turpentine.
Lavender:	the flowers are prescribed, in the popular medicine of the south of France, as being vermifuge, but have never been confirmed as such by our modern physicians
Lemon: (Ph)	stomach stimulant.
Mint:	carminative, stomach stimulant, specific against diarrhoea, colic, stomach cramps.
Neroli:	never prescribed for therapeutic purposes: orangeflower water is hypnotic for children, sedative and antispasmodic.
Rose:	never prescribed; if inhaled over a long period, it, like all essences, causes extremely severe migraines.[20]
Rosemary:	the leaves are used in infusions as a carminative and abortive in popular medicine.

Sage: (T, A)	the leaves are used as a stomach tonic, astringent against catarrh, diarrhoea.
Star anise:	stomachic, expectorant and carminative.
Thyme: (I)	disinfects the digestive tract, antispasmodic.
Wormwood: (T)	febrifuge, stimulates the stomach, vermifuge, abortive.
Yarrow:	against urine incontinence, gallstones, sedative and anti-gonorrhoeic.

Editor's Notes on oils

(C) = Carcinogenic (very low-level)
(I) = Irritant
(S) = Sensitiser (possibility of allergic reaction)
(T) = Toxic
(A) = Abortifacient
(Ph) = Photosensitizer (do not expose skin to UV rays after using this oil)

Some pure constituents are, on the other hand, held in slightly better regard:

Menthol:	excellent antiseptic and analgesic, depressive action on the nervous system, at low doses, paralyses voluntary movements at high doses, used as stomach stimulant, antiseptic, externally as antineuralgic and in inhalation as an antiseptic and decongestant.
Thymol:	internal antiseptic, specific against pleurisy, chronic bronchial catarrh, externally as a disinfectant.

These opinions are certainly not generally held, but whatever our admiration for Dr Reutter's work, we cannot help but notice the surprising paucity of information about essential oils.

It is against this background of ignorance about essential oils that we protest – a lack of knowledge which in our eyes is not altogether unintentional, and which must not be allowed to continue.

Chemically, essential oils are of enormous interest; pure constituents may sometimes be preferred, but their physiological action is always very significant and their potency often considerable. They deserve a proper place in pharmacopoeias for reasons which we will discuss later.

chapter four

MORE RECENT WORKS ON ESSENTIAL OILS

The sizeable bibliography of works on the therapeutic uses of essential oils testifies to the fact that modern schools have appealed against the somewhat summary judgement pronounced on essential oils in the last century.

Particularly over the last 50 years, the number of studies has multiplied, a situation not unrelated to our own early publications. In his bromatology studies (*Parfumerie Moderne* [Modern Perfumery], 1927), the pharmacist M. Renaudet gave the names of M. Calvello (1902), Marx (1903), K. Kobert (1906), R. Geinits (1912), O. Anselmino (1916), L. Clavel[21] (1918), S. Furukawa (1919) and J. R. Spinner (1920), all of whom should be added to the already impressive list of authors to whom we make reference in this book.

Before turning to this large body of literature, we feel we should summarise our own papers given at various conferences. They set the scene for new experiments which will need to be carried out on a larger scale.

Volatility and Odour are indicative of considerable physiological activity

This statement must form the basis of all work. Professor Raphaël Dubois' assertion that all volatile substances are anaesthetic should be borne in mind with regard to essential oils, a typical characteristic of which is volatility.[22]

We have tested many essential oils and substances, such as acetone, rarely used in general anaesthesia. All of them produced the pupillary reaction of dilation and fixity. While acetone, like ether, causes general anaesthesia, essential oils produce mainly local analgesia.

Intramuscular injections in massive doses have yielded interesting observations. We have used only oxidised aromatic substances or halogenated or nitrated compounds, with no terpenic hydrocarbons which do not enter the bloodstream and, like oil of turpentine, cause fixation abscesses. If, by accident or for as yet unexplained reasons, the terpene is not fixed, it particularly affects the bulb, causing symptoms of meningitis. When injecting massive doses of certain essences, allowance must be made for the actual mechanism of the normal fixation abscess; more consistent results may be obtained by using selected terpeneless oils, without a local abscess forming.

On the other hand, comparing the theory that fragrant emanations are material in nature – a theory supported by Fourcroy,

Berthollet, Hermann Boerhaave, Passy and others – with Becquerel and Durand's theory that emanations are corpuscular, or Heinrich Teudt's that scents are vibratory in nature, led us to develop a new hypothesis about the atomic composition of aromatic substances. This composition is what enables them to condense steam, as Durand noted in 1918, and is perhaps also the source of their therapeutic power. This hypothesis calls for in-depth study, but we thought it appropriate first to test the scale of the chemical function in relation to the physiological results obtained.

Thus far, these tests have covered aromatic constituents injected in their natural state, with neither a solvent nor a carrier substance, into the muscular mass. They were then conducted on the same products ingested via the digestive tract, first in their pure state, and then at various dilutions, particularly alcohol dilutions – the activity of the latter solutions being different, particularly in terms of bile reaction, because of the presence of alcohol.

The elimination of ingested aromatic substances begins within a few minutes, and that of injected substances within a matter of seconds (experiments on guinea pigs). If the animal is killed after a few minutes, the aromatic substances are found in any of the various elimination centres – liver, lung, kidney – and later in precise locations in the nervous centres depending upon the substances used.

GENERAL PROPERTIES OF CONSTITUENTS

To determine the possible applications of essential oils, we first studied the physical and chemical properties of the various aromatic constituents. The resulting observations are useful for the selection of essential oils which can be used in various circumstances and the avoidance of those which may not be indicated *a priori*.

Terpenes. Terpenes should be examined firstly as they are found in all essential oils to a greater or lesser degree. It was, incidentally, this study which led to our preference for the use of terpeneless essences and constituents for internal use.

Terpenes are light (density of 850/880 on average), have a relatively low boiling point (140/155°C at normal pressure), are only slightly soluble in dilute alcohol, are insoluble in water, soluble in benzene, ether, acetone and chloroform and only slightly soluble in liquid potassium soaps.

Terpenes oxidise readily, especially in the presence of water. In nature, they oxidise gradually as the aromatic substances rise into the uppermost organs of the plants. Essences extracted from wood contain more terpenes than those from leaves, which, in turn, contain more than those extracted from flowers.[23]

A good example of this is pine. While its resin contains only terpenes and colophony, its leaves contain borneol, terpineol and ethers of these alcohols, which are the oxidation products of primitive pinene.

Terpenes oxidise rapidly and extensively. This property is used in paints made of oil and essence. Oil of turpentine fixes the oxygen on the oxidisable products (linolein and gums) and produces the glazed finish.

Cases of rapid, spontaneous oxidation, with heating and ignition, are not at all rare: this is what causes cleaning rags to catch on fire in perfume factories, and sometimes causes fires to break out in pine forests during tapping.[24].

Oxidation is often so considerable that ozone forms. The antiseptic power of terpenes vaporised in the air is often attributed to this property.

The following study on eucalyptus essence shows that the crude essence, which contains terpenes and a small amount of water from distillation, is more active than pure eucalyptol[25] which lacks chemical oxidizing activity, and an initial analysis of its chemical formula reveals its neutrality.

Terpenes have an interesting revulsive[26] effect on the epidermis, the applications of which we will highlight.

Terpenes can therefore be used, to a certain extent, as volatile air antiseptics. They can be used instead of pinene on fixation abscesses, provided that the mechanism of such abscesses continues to be understood as it is today. Limonene is a more active substance than pinene. Taken internally, terpenes dissolve mucous, damage the stomach lining, cause auto-digestion, ulcerations and painful irritation.[27] The accidental absorption of terpenes by a dog resulted in bloody faeces.

The reputation most essences have of being caustic or toxic is due to the presence of terpenes and their irritant action. The removal of these hydrocarbons transforms the action of essences.[28]

REGARDING THE CONSTITUENTS OF EUCALYPTUS ESSENCE

In the *Pharmaceutical Journal*, M. E.-M. Holmes summarised the work of Baker and Smith and that of E. Hall and A. Walsch at the Sydney Laboratory of Physiology. As eucalyptus essences are often sold with a guaranteed eucalyptol content – a substance with no apparent activity[29] – it is appropriate to mention these works here as they are a fine example of the sort of errors which can be made (and in some cases perpetuated for a considerable time) by inadequate examination of the facts.

These scientists demonstrated that phellandrene is one of the major constituents of eucalyptus essences and that piperitone and aromadendral are also highly active substances from the bactericidal and physiological viewpoint.

M. Hall Euthbert points out that of the twenty-two constituents found to date in essences of eucalyptus, eucalyptol is the one which was – wrongly – attributed with therapeutic value. This is because the physiological effects of ethers and oxides have only recently been discovered.

Certain constituents found either in small quantities or only in certain oils do not seem to have any great therapeutic value. Others disappear at rectification or are so irritating that they cannot be administered with impunity. The constituents of interest in eucalyptus essences are above all: eudesmol, aromadendral, piperitone and aromadendrene, d-pinene, l-pinene and phellandrene.

To the great surprise of those conducting the experiments, they found that pure eucalyptol, containing only a trace of pinene, had poor antiseptic qualities, less than the other constituents. It was later realised that the bactericidal power of eucalyptol varied depending on its ozone and catalyser content, such as acetic acid and iron or the copper dissolved in it.

Essences containing aromadendrene (*E. Hemiphloia*) are the most bactericidal. Next come those containing piperitone, eudesmol and phellandrene. These compounds release only a small quantity of ozone and this is released only because it is impossible to remove all the terpenes completely.

Thus, the presence of ozone is due to terpenes: when phellandrene and aromadendrene are exposed to the air on starched potassium iodide paper, the blue coloration does not appear immediately; instead the reaction takes place after 20 to 30 minutes and the terpenes resinify. Phellandrene and aromadendrene ozonise more rapidly than d-pinene, and d-pinene more rapidly than l-pinene. According to M. Hall, the variable quantities of ozone found in eucalyptol and in rectified essences is explained by the presence of variable quantities of pinene in the crude essences.

The conclusions of the experiments are as follows:

Eucalyptol, except when charged with ozone, is the least anti-septic of the constituents.

The terpenes are the source of the ozone, and the constituents which ozonise most easily in eucalyptus essences are phellandrene and aromadendral.

It would be worthwhile including a test for ozone identification in eucalyptus essences in the pharmacopoeia.

Piperitone and the essences in which it is found seem to be of greater interest. The author has observed acute cases of influenza and coryza improved by piperitone from essences of *Eucalyptus Dives* or *E. radiata*, often confused with *E. Amygdalina*. Piperitone acts as an anaesthetic and vasoconstrictor but differs from menthol in that it acts on sensitive nerves: placed on the tongue, it first creates a hot sharp sensation followed by a feeling of freshness and numb-ness. It increases salivation and has a stimulating and carminative effect. In frogs, it first acts as a general stimulant, then paralyses the central nervous system and the respiration, but has only a slight action on the heart.

The action of eucalyptus leaf infusions on glycosuria indicates that there is a larger quantity of the active substance in the leaves of *E. Globulus* than in those of *E. Punctata*. The action of this same infusion against malaria cannot yet be attributed to a known substance.

These observations should completely overturn specialists' views on eucalyptus essences. When used as disinfectants, they should not be completely dehydrated,'[30] the containers should be plugged only with cotton wool, which is permeable to air. Also, coloured glass containers should not be used as the essence should be exposed to light.[31]

This same type of study could be conducted on most essential oils.

THE PROPERTIES OF AROMATIC ALCOHOLS

Alcohols are the most numerous and most abundant constituents of essences. They have a higher density than terpenes
(870 to 930) and are partially soluble in water – 10 to 40 centigrams
per litre on average, sometimes more. They are very soluble in weak
alcohol (except in sesquiterpenic alcohols) and in all proportions in
strong alcohol, and are also readily soluble in soap solutions. They
have an intense action, are easily absorbed and non-irritating and
diffuse rapidly when injected in muscle.

Particular mention should be made here of borneol, an alcohol
or camphor from the *Dryobalanops* of Borneo, no longer held in the
regard it deserves in Europe. In its ether form, crystallised borneol
liquefies. We have used it successfully to combat serious cases of
septicaemia in veterinary practice.

Borneol is not as strong a vasoconstrictor as menthol, but it is
toxic and not very tonic, even in doses much higher than those
allowed for menthol. Borneol was the first of the two to become
known and was considered a panacea. A recent archeological find in
Italy led to the discovery of organic substances which had been
perfectly preserved for at least 2,000 years in a vase containing
borneol or camphor of Borneo. Camphor of Japan, which is a
ketone (and thus one of the most toxic of constituents),[32] is a
completely different substance, with properties almost the opposite
of those of borneol.

In 923, Rhazes spoke of camphor from the Greater Islands
(Sunda and Sumatra), where only *Dryobalanops camphora* grows.
It was marvellously effective against the plague. Schroeder's
Pharmacopoeia of 1698, Volume I, states that there is no more
prodigious an alexipharmac.[33] Heinsius, a doctor from Verona, had
concocted an anti-plague oil containing amber (which, through
distillation, also yields borneol) and camphor of Borneo. His cures
were so spectacular that the city erected a triumphal column in his
honour.

Kampfer (1690) stated that camphor of Borneo was among the
most precious merchandise exported to Japan by the Dutch. In 636,
it was mentioned along with musk, ambergris and sandalwood as
being among the treasures that Khosro II, King of Persia, possessed
in the Nadain palace on the Tigris in Babylon. At the time of the fall
of Khalife Fatinite Mostanser in Cairo in the second century, Arab

historians mentioned censers of camphor decorated with gold and precious stones. It was also made into pomanders and sachets against the plague well before camphor of Japan (ketone of *Laurus camphora*) was imported. This caused confusion which favoured camphor simply because of its similarity in appearance and odour. Ketonic camphor is currently used in immense quantities, largely due to the reputation of camphor of Borneo.

Yet while borneol is aphrodisiac, tonic, stimulating and highly antiseptic, ketonic camphor, like all ketones, is anaphrodisiac, tranquillising and toxic.[34] This confusion on the part of European doctors is not found among Orientals, who remain loyal to alcoholic camphor (borneol) but look unfavourably on ketonic camphor, or at least restrict its use.

The essences of rosemary, sage, pine and fir contain borneol and its ethers. This is what gives them their strong antiseptic qualities and accounts for their medicinal applications. Essence of rosemary is considered a beneficial stomachic against atonic dyspepsia. The leaf infusion is stimulating and has yielded excellent results for some feverish conditions causing temporary but worrying prostration.

Cazin obtained marvellous results for pernicious bouts of malaria. Brissemoret, in his *Essais sur les préparations galéniques* [Essays on galenical preparations], lists it as a stimulant and tonic because of the presence of borneol along with camphor, cineol, pinene and camphene. It is a vermifuge and an emmenagogue.

Sage, recommended by Van Swieten, also combats sweating in the feverish. Trousseau, Pidoux and Gubier recommended it as a restorative tonic. Chapoutot attempted to show the therapeutic properties of *Salvia salvatrix naturea conciliatrix* sage, as did the Salernitan School, which considered it a panacea.

Terpineol, also common in many essences, is similar to terpine hydrate in terms of physiological activity. It is decongestant and Americans attribute to it a number of interesting properties which need verification. Terpineol is also found in essence of juniper, together with a very high proportion of terpenes, which is why Reutter simply classes it with oil of turpentine.

Linalol is found in many essential oils either in the form of alcohol (essence of rosewood) or esters,[35] such as bergamot and lavender. The properties of these two essences show that much can be expected of this alcohol. In orangeflower absolute, which, thanks to the interesting works of Grégoire, is known to have a hypnotic effect at low doses, linalol is found together with methyl anthranilate, which may be the decisive factor in its highly specific action, rather than the linalol itself. Clary sage, which has a reputation as a panacea dating from antiquity, is also principally composed of linalol and its acetate. However, the substances of an, as yet, unknown nature, found in small quantities in this essence may also explain its particular action.[36]

In our tests, we have found that linalol, terpineol and geraniol seem to be more anaesthetic than borneol although, in general, alcohol injections are always more painful than injections of the esters of these alcohols. Alcohols are diuretic and are eliminated in part via the kidney and in part via the lungs. A 1 cm^3 dose per 500-gram animal did not produce any sign of intoxication. The fatal dose is generally 3 to 4 grams, with death generally occurring by asphyxia: the lungs, saturated with the essential oil being eliminated, dehydrate and cease to function. Thus, strictly speaking, there is no toxicity. If elimination through the respiratory tract occurs quickly enough to avoid asphyxia, fixation is observed on the nervous centres, very rarely to the point of hemiplegia. But here again, this can be attributed to a physical phenomenon of fatty matter being dissolved by a solvent – the 3-gram dose for a 500-gram animal is no longer medicinal.

THE PROPERTIES OF AROMATIC ETHERS

E thers seem to act largely via their acid: ethers from the same acid combined with different alcohols present reactions characteristic of the acid and not of the alcohol. Esters readily produce epileptiform spasms.[37] At a dose of 3 grams per kilogram,[38] death occurs due to heart failure. In autopsy, the acetates are often found accumulated in the gall bladder. Formates accelerate the heartbeat and, at high doses, provoke paralysis of the hind quarters and the diaphragm. Benzoates are eliminated primarily via the kidneys and the lungs, thus confirming the disinfectant properties of metallic benzoates. Butyrates are easily eliminated via the lungs and kidneys, even at a dose of 2 to 3 grams per kilogram, without incident. Essence of lavender, the esters of which are a mixture of linalyl acetate and linalyl butyrate, tends to give the reaction of the butyrates. Since, in analysis, the proportion of butyrate seems low, one can say that a small quantity of butyric acid is sufficient to mask the action of the acetic acid, but, here again, our tests took us far beyond medicinal doses, since essential oils become effective at extremely low doses, in the order of milligrams per animal kilo-gram. Action at homeopathic doses has formed the subject of some interesting studies: essence of mint in toothpaste seems to cancel out the effect of medication whereas aniseed oil does not have this disadvantage. Benzyl benzoate[39] is antispasmodic. Spasmodic con-stipation, uterine colic, bronchial spasms and persistant hiccups cannot withstand 10 to 30 drops per day of an alcoholic solution to the 5th centesimal (*Presse médicale* [Medical Press], Oct. 1920). Whooping cough is much improved. Heart problems abate under this substance which has a hypotensive action without affecting the kidney. This substance eases angina pectoris and arterial hyperten-sion better than sodium nitrate, even where the patient no longer reacts to the latter (Macht of Baltimore).

THE PROPERTIES OF AROMATIC ALDEHYDES

Aldehydes are highly effective antiseptics and can be categorised, in this respect, very closely to phenols although they do not have their caustic property.

Cinnamic aldehyde is almost as effective as eugenol, with which it is found in a number of volatile oils. It is analgesic and, when used to treat pain, often produces results similar to those of methyl salicylate or essence of wintergreen – although it does not smell noticeably more pleasant. The planters and indigenous peoples of the Pacific Islands often use it for this purpose. Distilled cinnamon water has also been used for dressings and for treating stomach ulcers. Cabanès (*Bull. Gén. de thér.* [General Therapy Journal]) states that cinnamon essence destroys *Eberthella typhosa* in just 12 minutes. The antiseptic properties of essences, however well proven they may be, are but one aspect of the matter under study.

Galangal (*Alpinia galanga*), the principal constituent of which is methyl cinnamate, acts primarily via its cinnamic acid; and, as mentioned in the previous section, the acids of the ethers have a dominant action. It is thus not surprising that Confucius recom-mends this drug, which the Chinese call Chiang, and sees it as a panacea.

Citral is really only known for its deodorant powers, yet it has other qualities too. Benzoic aldehyde is little used. It converts rapidly into benzoic acid, which has properties of which greater use could be made in culinary and confectionery preparations.

THE PROPERTIES OF AROMATIC KETONES

Ketones are considered toxic, and our tests partially confirm previous literature. The ketones in artemisia essence[40] are abortive, states Doctor Lestrat in his thesis on *Juniperus phoenica*.

Simon and Mitscherlich state that essence of fennel is toxic because of its fenchone[41] and indeed we have seen livers turned brown due to the repeated ingestion of fennel solution. Star anise and anise, which contain only anethol, are thus to be recommended as a substitute. While fenchone is not readily eliminated via the rectum, anethol is easily eliminated in this way. Essence of caraway produces ketone-specific symptoms caused by carvone.[41] The legal provisions against absinthe containing essence of wormwood are thus justified, at least insofar as French essences of wormwood contain thujone. Terpenes should always be removed from essence of mint which, in its raw state, contains menthone, as menthone is eliminated during fractionation along with the terpenes, which have a similar boiling point.

Ketonic essences are not, however, totally without merit. Essences of artemisia heal sores, prevent fatigue, are antispasmodic and emmenagoguic. Those of yarrow are anti-epileptic stomachics and used in large quantities in the preparation of vermouths. *Achillea moschata* is used in infusions against chills and sudden indispositions. In the Italian Alps, *Achillea clavennae* is used to aid respiration at high mountain altitudes. *Achillea ageratum* is used as an expectorant and stomachic. *Achillea ptarmica*, with a taste reminiscent of tarragon, activates salivation and heals toothache. It is also used against epilepsy.

Achillea herba rota is sudorific. Murtih attests that he has seen it cure pleurisy when used in the first days of the illness. Yarrow flowers – also known as "nose-bleed" – cause nasal haemorrhaging and heal sores and toothache. Yarrow tea heals haemorrhoids.

In Savoy, says Chabert, caraway, coriander and fennel are considered emmenagogues. First they were made into virus oils, then liqueurs. At homeopathic doses, ketonic essences are very active, as expected in view of their relative toxicity.

The Properties of Aromatic Phenols

Phenols are the strongest of the aromatic bactericides. They are highly soluble: water dissolves up to 1 gram per litre, and liquid soaps up to 40 grams per litre (soap containing 30% fatty acids). They have the disadvantage of being slightly caustic,[42] but infinitely less so than the phenols (phenic acid) or cresols extracted from coal distillates. They do not burn tissue, but do not have the cytophylactic power of other essential oil constituents.

This is why aromatic phenols can be used only at lower doses than other substances. Eugenol yields excellent results in dental surgery and is already replacing p-cresol-based compounds, for which it should always be substituted either alone or mixed with geraniol or citronellol.

J. Cloquet reports that when the Dutch destroyed the clove trees on the Island of Ternate in the Moluccas archipelago, the colony was decimated by several epidemic diseases never previously observed. This is evidence that the mere emanations of clove leaves and flowers suffice to purify the air.

Uses of thymol as an intestinal disinfectant and vermifuge are well known. Di-iodothymol also enjoyed widespread popularity for a time. Today, preference is given to carvacrol which, while having the same properties, is less caustic than thymol. Carvacrol is better eliminated via the respiratory tract.

Carvacrol-based rubs, embrocations and revulsives offer undeniable relief from illnesses of the respiratory track. We will look at this new mode of applying essential oils and their absorption through the skin in a subsequent chapter.

Doctor Forgues, who is often mentioned in this study and who has had numerous opportunities to treat impoverished natives in Morocco and Tunisia, has time and again used an inexpensive and effective scented preparation, *Zit ou Zââter*, that is, oil and thyme, two readily available products. A decoction of fresh or dried thyme in olive oil is applied in compresses to the natives' sores, which are often phagedenic. The results have always been satisfactory.

Essence of wild thyme, which contains carvacrol, is already used for intratracheal injections in the form of vegetable oils mixed with essential oils (Balvay pneumobiol).

This small amount of information about "constituents" shows why it is essential to be well aware of the composition of essential oils and to use the pure constituents whenever the presence of a rare constituent or one which is difficult to isolate would not lend guaranteed specific properties to the essential oil.

REASONS FOR FAILURE IN THE THERAPEUTIC USE OF COMMERCIAL ESSENCES

The complexity of essential oils and the differences observable in their centesimal composition, due either to their origin, the distillation process or any number of other causes mean the practitioner must diligently monitor the substances he uses, the principal constants of which must be carefully verified in order to ensure consistent therapeutic effects.

We have already seen the surprises eucalyptus essence holds in store and, in fact, nearly all commercial crude essential oils have the same disadvantages. Even analyses in pharmacopoeias are for the most part inadequate. Thus, as medicinal applications increase in number, minimum and maximum chemical and physical indices for the products to be used should be established.

Hitherto, the presence of various quantities of terpenes in the essences used has been the cause of a large number of failures for we have observed that the properties of terpenes are highly particular and stand in the way of positive results far more often than one might imagine.[43]

Adulteration of the so-called veterinary spike lavender essence with turpentine oil, which is a terpene (pinene), is the main reason for the gradual abandonment of this product, despite its previously acknowledged action. Although the application of highly pure spike essence has been demonstrated to promote the healing of animal sores, new fur growth, the rapid healing of scabies and ringworm, it is no less true that the use of spike essence mixed with turpentine causes itching and eczema without giving the desired relief.

Whereas the use of terpeneless essence of lavender gives immediate results, that of a non-rectified essential oil is far from satisfactory. We were informed of this recently, with regard to a case of furunculosis, where terpeneless essences healed the condition perfectly the first time but the application of crude oil resulted in no improvement when used for a relapse.

The use of essences of mint containing a ketone (menthone) can be unsatisfactory. The use of crude essence of lemongrass containing methylheptenone is less indicated than the terpeneless essence from which it has been removed. Essences of lemon, orange and bergamot, which still contain non-volatile substances also extracted by the hand or machine method, can have disappointing results.[44]

In any case, crude essential oils are hardly soluble in water and only slightly miscible with liquid soaps. They are often used with fatty excipients which insulate the mucous membranes or sores from contact with the air, which must be avoided for numerous reasons.[45]

The high solubility of terpeneless essences is demonstrated by the following examples. 9 to 10 parts of 90% alcohol are needed to dissolve one part of essence of angelica; the terpeneless essence is soluble at any proportion in the same solvent. Its solubility is therefore at least ten times greater.

50 parts of 70% alcohol are needed to dissolve one part of petitgrain essence. Two and a half parts of alcohol of the same strength are sufficient to dissolve one part of the terpeneless essence. Its solubility is thus twenty times greater. The solubility of coriander essence is also increased tenfold, that of lemon, orange and juniper even more so, that of most other volatile essences is multiplied by 5 or 10.

Glycerine dissolves appreciable quantities of terpeneless essences.

This solubility can be of enormous benefit. Doctor Forgues cites an interesting case. A young girl suffering from a serious stomach ulcer after ingesting sulphuric acid was not able to alleviate her gastric problems with mint alcohol, for instance, which caused dreadful pain. Mint-leaf tea did not have a sufficiently strong action and milk produced acid gases which irritated the oesophageal burns. Cold water, perfumed with terpeneless mint essence relieved the distension of her stomach, thus allowing her to recover properly in a short time. A stomach ulcer which could not tolerate an alcohol fennel tincture was likewise healed with extemporaneous fennel water obtained by beating the terpeneless essence in water. The sugary granules of essences means that up to 1 gram of terpeneless essence can be dissolved per litre under certain conditions.

Extemporaneous aromatic waters can be used for intramuscular and intravenous injection without any risk of flocculation or mishap. Glycerine ovules containing sufficient quantities of essences can be prepared without the need for any special solvent.

VITAMINS AND ESSENCES

T wenty years ago Funk and G. Hopkins declared that certain substances absorbed by animals through the digestive tract in very small quantities are absolutely essential to the development of the organism and the maintenance of life.

There are two groups of vitamins: those soluble in fats and fatty solvents, and those soluble in water. The first are called A, D and E, and the second B and C.

According to Kathleen Culhane and S. W. F. Underhill (Chemist and Druggist, Feb. 1933), vitamin A is an anti-infectious vitamin. It prevents mucous cells from keratinising and being vulnerable to invasion by microorganisms. In this respect, it is comparable to many essential oils which have the same property and even give cells a remarkable ability to proliferate while destroying infectious bacteria.

From the chemical perspective, vitamin A is a saturated alcohol with the empirical formula $C^{20}H^{30}$. Those vitamins which it has been possible to prepare to a certain degree of purity appear in the form of a pale yellow viscous liquid, stable to heat, without the presence of oxygen and resistant to alkalis. Acids and other reactives act by destroying the double bond of the molecule. This vitamin is found in fresh vegetables and in milk, butter and egg yolk, which in turn probably obtain it from the vegetable matter on which the animals feed.

Carotene, which generally accompanies vitamin A and converts to this vitamin in the body, following reactions that occur in digestion, has the formula $C^{40}H^{56}$. It encompasses two geranial rings connected by a long isopropene chain (Y.R.N. *Parfums de France* [Perfumes of France], April 1932) and resembles beta-ionone.

Lycopene, found in tomatoes, appears to be the corresponding aliphatic hydrocarbon (Karrer and Bachmann), and carotene would appear to derive from it by cyclisation of the type: pseudo-ionone, ionone beta. On the basis of the study of its oxidation, xanthophyll, a substance almost as common as carotene, is also a cyclo-geranial derivative. It is a $C^{40}H^{56}O^2$ alcohol.

Chlorophyll is always found with carotene and xanthophyll, the relative proportions of these two substances varying within a narrow range, and consists of an association of a colorant and phytol.[46]

Phytol is a $C^{20}H^{30}OH$ ethylene alcohol: 2, 6, 10, 14-

tetramethylhexadecene-14-ol-16 (K. F. Gottwald Fischer). It is thus an aliphatic octa-hydro-diterpene alcohol, which was made synthetically by G. Fottwald Fisher and Kûrt Lôwenberg from the pseudo-ionone.

Lycopene can derive from two phytol molecules by bonding or dehydrogenation. It thus seems to have a genetic relationship to phytol, carotene and xanthophyll, and also an undeniable association with certain terpene alcohols.

Extracts rich in vitamin A, treated with ozone, have produced geranial acids, β-ionone oxidation products similar to those of carotene.

One of the most fascinating areas of current scientific progress (Y.R.N.) is thus the synthesis of substances in the β-ionone group, similar in structure to carotene, and research into their vitamin activity.

Vitamin D, which plays an important role in calcification and, if lacking from children's food, results in skeletal deformation and poor dentition, was obtained from ergosterol by exposing the latter to rays of less than 320 p.p.: the vitamin forms on human skin by the action of solar radiation. It is an isomer alcohol of ergosterol, with the formula $C^{28}H^{44}O$: it is resistant to alkalis and relatively stable in the presence of acids or when exposed to oxygen and heat.

Bourdillon and Windaus each obtained it independently, the former in the crystallised state and his name for it, "calciferol", was adopted. Ergosterol is one of the substances which Abderhalen called sterols. These are substances which contain an alcohol hydroxyl and which, when heated with sodic lime, do not yield fatty acids of the same carbon condensation, as do aliphatic alcohols. With digitonin, sterols generally produce addition compounds from which they can be regenerated.

Ergosterol $C^{27}H^{42}O$, one of the most common sterols, has an alcohol function and three double bonds, which allows a number of isomers to exist. The isomer considered a vitamin does not produce a compound with digitonin, nor the Diels-Adler reaction with maleic or citraconic anhydride. To prepare vitamin D, irradiated yeast is extracted from ergosterol and treated cold with citraconic anhydride; the non-compound part is crystallised in aqueous acetone.

Skin readily absorbs vitamin D, which literally "rejuvenates" it. This substance will therefore grow in importance in the field of cosmetics.

Vitamins act at infinitesimal doses. Recent tests by Dr Sassard using lavender essence in a highly dilute state seem to show that essential oils also act at very low doses. Other essential oils with a composition more similar to that of vitamins will probably yield convincing results at even lower doses. However, a major consideration in favour of essential oils is the fact that they are totally safe. Vitamin D becomes toxic at a dose of 9.04 milligrams, whereas essential oils present practically no danger at all.[47] Perhaps then, the partnership of vitamins and essences will result in another form of use in which essences act as antitoxic substances.

Vitamin D abuse can cause massive calcification and acute lesions of the kidney. Since it is easy to choose an essential oil which counters this property, safe active ingredients could perhaps be obtained in this way. However, intravenous injections of aromatic waters frequently lead to a hardening of the vein walls.

Essences which have the properties of both hormones and vitamins truly merit the attention of practitioners (Aschheim and Holweg in the *Dt. Med. Wochenschr.* [German Medical Weekly], 1933, page 12).

Might this connection between vitamins and certain aromatic constituents serve to explain the curious activity of the latter, particularly their prodigious ability to activate tissue and renew cell proliferation, to produce fully restored tissue where there have been large losses of substance and, for example, to heal, without apparent scarring, burns which, if treated with other substances, would leave distressing disfigurements? Further work in this area will enable us to clarify this question.

In any case, the parallel we have just drawn between vitamins and essential oils shows that the defensive powers of tissue against attack by microorganisms does not depend only on the antiseptic or sterilising power of the remedies used. Although essences do possess the highest level of this bactericidal power, and no substance currently used in surgery or medicine can rival them in this regard (especially when one considers the effect of traditional antiseptics on tissue), it does seem that we should pay attention not only to the sterilising effect of aromatic substances, but also to properties they have which are similar to those of vitamins.

Essential oils diluted to a degree at which they no longer have any effect on cultures in vitro, still have a clear, rapid and beneficial action on the living body.*

---

* This phenomenon has been confirmed recently by doctors in France, and may be due to an immuno-stimulant effect.

chapter five

AROMATHERAPY

The chemical properties and compositions of essential oils cover all the known chemical "functions". They should therefore be suitable for use in widely divergent situations. At present, only a very small number of constituents is known and used therapeutically, yet there is no reason why worthwhile applications should not be found for them all, used internally and externally.

While the essential oils suggested most often hitherto presented a certain number of disadvantages such as:

1. insolubility in water, glycerine and solvents other than concentrated alcohol, ether, benzene etc.,
2. poor keeping qualities due to the presence of oxidisable terpenes,
3. unstable composition (due to the very nature of the substances extracted from plants subjected to harsh weather conditions) etc.,

the pure constituents, on the other hand, keep well, are relatively pure and very stable. Terpeneless essences, which have the same properties as the constituents, may be used to preserve the power of "mixtures of oxygenated constituents" formed by certain natural essential oils.

Indeed, it has been noted, in the study of the sterilising power of essential oils, that mixtures of constituents have a greater effect than the same constituents working individually. We can therefore assume *a priori* that, in nature and otherwise, the total power of mixtures of aromatic constituents is greater than the sum of the power of the individual parts.[48] As long as certain essential oils have "unknown constituents" or constituents which are difficult to isolate, but which appear to have valuable properties, it will be worthwhile using these essential oils in their fully terpeneless state.

Terpeneless essences are readily soluble in all kinds of media; they keep well, their composition can be easily checked, their therapeutic action is clear and constant and the absence of terpenes is an indisputable benefit.

The weaknesses of crude essential oils are certainly the primary reason for their rejection and the justifiable suspicion with which they have been viewed hitherto. Thanks to modern production techniques, essential oils can now be made which are pure enough for medical purposes. These diverse substances already have an undeniable action in a wide range of circumstances: all that remains for us to do is to widen the scope of experimentation.

ACTION OF ESSENCES ON THE RESPIRATORY TRACT

Numerous findings have already been made in this regard. Because of their volatile nature and the ease with which they can be introduced into the respiratory tract as vapours, essential oils have often been recommended for treating diseases of the respiratory organs.

Wet inhalations use mixed "water-essence" vapours at less than 100 degrees centigrade. Unfortunately, at this temperature, the action of steam cannot always be reconciled with the treatment intended. For this reason, certain devices have been invented which enable pure vapours to be obtained from essences or alternatively a state of division comparable to gases.

Dr Forgues states that, in these conditions, the absorption of essential oils accelerates respiratory movement and increases its range with a subsequent effect on the heart and the circulation.

As early as 1906, Dr Couëtoux de Blain, to avoid using hot, wet vapours, treated bronchial diseases with dry inhalations by evaporating or burning certain aromatic mixtures on a heated iron spoon. He recommended the following mixtures:

Expectorant mixture:

Essence of elecampane	1 gr.
" of juniper	3 grs
" of melissa	2 "
" of sage	1 "

Balsamic mixture:

Essence of eucalyptus	4 grs
" of wild thyme	2 "
" of hyssop	2 "
" of cubeb	2 "

Sedative mixture:

Essence of sage	3 grs
" of marjoram	2 "
" of mint	2 "
" of meadowsweet	0.40

Other mixtures can of course also be imagined which could be used in a course of treatment for all respiratory diseases, by monitoring the progress of the disease and using the appropriate mixture for the patient's state:

Antipyogenic[49] mixture:
Essence of wild thyme .... 3 grs
    "   of lavender .... 2 "
    "   of cinnamon .... 1 "
    "   of rosemary .... 4 "

Vulnerary[50] mixture:
Essence of lavender .... 5 grs
    "   of verbena .... 1 "
    "   of mint .... 1 "
    "   of Cedar of Lebanon .... 3 "

Antispasmodic mixture:
Essence of cypress .... 5 grs
    "   of Norwegian pine .... 1 "
    "   of cajeput .... 4 "

Decongestant mixture:
Essence of mint .... 4 grs
    "   of *Eucalyptus dives* .... 3 "
Pure borneol .... 3 "

Siccatives mixture:
Essence of niaouli .... 5 grs
    "   of geranium .... 2 "
d-terpineol .... 3 "

These various preparations, either vaporised in boiling water or dissolved in volatile solvents and evaporated in a bowl of water, can be used to treat asthma, simple head colds, bronchitis, whooping cough and inflammatory or bacterial diseases. The nature and the number of inhalations will vary at the discretion of the physician in attendance.

The use of terpeneless essences prevents the irritation caused by the absorption of terpenes. The greatest benefit can be obtained from terpenes in wet vapours for, in such conditions, terpenes partially ozonise, thus increasing their antiseptic power (Baker and Smith). If not only a bactericidal action is wanted, vulnerary essences or, in some cases, constituents which stimulate or inhibit secretions can be used. Cypress essence, considered to be antispasmodic, is of benefit in treating whooping cough. It has long been used in Germany and with a certain reticence in France, but it has always produced favourable results.

Wild thyme is more frequently used; it is recommended in popular medicine. Dr A. Balvay uses it in an oily composition (pneumobiol) for intratracheal injection (*Paris médical*, 1921). It produces a sensation of euphoria, alleviates dyspnoea and therefore effects a positive change in the patient's haematosis disorder and normalises physiological organ function. Breathlessness is practically eliminated and the sputum of tuberculosis patients is more fluid, thus easing expectoration. Tuberculosis patients gain weight and their general condition improves. The use of essences is not indicated in cases of haemoptysis.[52]

Dr Ferrua states that *Inula helenium L.*[53] essence makes guinea pigs resistant to the tubercle bacillus and that this essence merits further study.

Synthetic products to be recommended include certain cresol ethers. In the Middle Ages, a goat was kept near consumptives. It was said that the strong smell of the goat chased away the pathogens. We should never simply dismiss traditions without attempting to understand their underlying meaning. We produced, synthetically, the odour of goat (metacresyl phenylacetate). On the basis of its composition, this substance seems to be a powerful antiseptic for the respiratory tract. The smells of cowsheds or stables were considered healthy in past centuries and today a pleasant form of their essential principles can be reproduced from other p- or o-cresyl phenylacetates or from coumarin, methylumbelliferone or methylhydroquinones, together with labiate essences.[54]

Dr Forgues also advocates certain essences for the treatment of diphtheria. During a serious diphtheria epidemic in 1912 (with a mortality rate of 13%), at a time when serotherapy was already widely practised, he decided to try making a wash with an aromatic mixture intended to replace mouthwashes made from salicyclic acid, methylene blue or sodium borate. He adopted the following preparation:

Terpeneless lavender essence:
    "   thyme essence
    "   rose essence   }   3 grs each
Artificial violet

Alcohol 95° q.s. to dissolve
neutral glycerine
$\left.\vphantom{\begin{matrix}a\\b\end{matrix}}\right\}$ 100 grs

The results were extremely satisfactory. In one family with three cases at the same time, one patient was treated with mentholated methylene blue mouthwash, another with a mouthwash made from the essences listed above and the third with a throat wash made from the same oils. The third patient healed most quickly both locally and generally. Pain when swallowing soon disappeared. The "membrane" quickly changed from grey to white and the nauseating odour, specific to some types of diphtheria, soon abated. Serotherapy had, of course, been used in all three cases.

In other cases, this doctor also noticed the rapid disappearance of dysphagia and the unpleasant smell of gangrenous abscesses or imminent phlegmon common in malignant anginas.

G. Renaudet states that the essences of aniseed, star aniseed, cypress, eucalyptus, sage and turpentine may always be used as expectorants. Dr Reynier proposed sodium cinnamate which, according to our studies, acts primarily via its cinnamic acid. According to his report to the Académie de Médecine, Dr Reynier had successfully tried sodium cinnamate in his practice in Lariboisière, administering subcutaneous injections of eight to fifteen centigrams every other day.[55]

With this method, M. Reynier and two of his colleagues achieved rapid improvement and even complete recovery in several cases of tuberculosis.

By his tests, O. Soltmann (1904) established the resolvent action of eucalyptus, cypress and mint essences on the mucous membranes of the nose and throat (nasopharynx) and the respiratory tract.

O. Anselmino claims that burnet, used in popular medicine for coughs and hoarseness, acts via its essential oil.

Essence of cedar of Lebanon,[56] a balsamic used for bacterial infections of the urinary tract, is also effective in treating respiratory diseases (Renaudet).

Geranium is wonderfully effective in the treatment of certain painful mouth and pharyngeal ailments, mouth ulcers, acute stomatitis and minor throat infections (Dr P. Jucquelier).

Mint essence is analgesic, deodorant and antiseptic. The oily solution of menthol is used in mouthwashes for the vocal chords, in intranasal instillations and in tracheal injections, as well as being used as an anti-emetic to prevent vomiting in tuberculosis patients.

However, for internal use, old preparations of powdered mint are preferable (Dr P. Jucquelier).

For diseases of the respiratory organs, five drops of hyssop essence on sugar are administered (Bull. Schimmel, April–May, 1905). In other cases, it is helpful to administer the remedy in the form of gelatine capsules (A. Sassard). Bitter orange essence is said to be good for singers.

AROMATIC REVULSION

Cutaneous absorption of aromatic products in the preventive or curative treatment of pulmonary ailments.

We have particularly focused on the revulsive based on essence of wild thyme which we invented in 1918 and which produces such good results, particularly in preventing pulmonary accidents following narcosis and in healing all bronchial and lung ailments. This revulsive not only causes significant local vasodilation and stimulates peripheral circulation, but is also the source of genuine cutaneous absorption of aromatic substances which then work not only on the part of the skin where the revulsive is applied, but also inside the body.

In an article published in 1932 in *Le Progrès Médical* [Medical Progress], Dr Loeper reviewed the medicines and the absorption channels used in cases of pulmonary antisepsis. In this otherwise comprehensive study, cutaneous absorption was hardly mentioned and almost immediately rejected as largely impractical and even dangerous at times.

"It appeared to us," says Dr Sassard, "that this means of absorption did not merit such ostracism and that, without wishing to generalise its use, it was, to the contrary, the best channel to use in many specific cases."

If we examine the methods currently used to introduce antiseptic medicines into the system during chronic or acute pulmonary ailments, we can see that there are some which are only used occasionally, such as Rosenthal's intra- or trans-tracheal injections or the endovenous introduction of antiseptic substances. Other methods, such as introducing medicinal substances into the pleura (Lemaire), are so new that no assessment is possible.

There are, therefore, the following methods:

1. Inhalations and variations thereof; vapour treatments or sprays. This method gives excellent results when used for the upper respiratory tract but does have certain disadvantages for pulmonary ailments. As Loeper himself notes, an inhalation is irritating if it contains alcohol and pure balsamic products and, furthermore, inhalations do not usually penetrate deeply enough.

2. Hypodermic or intramuscular injections. This method is widely used and has many advantages but cannot be used indiscriminately and requires the presence of a doctor or a trained ancillary. Finally, despite improvements, many of these solutions are either irritants or their reabsorption is too slow.

3. The gastric tract is most commonly used, but wrongly so in our opinion. The only advantage of this method is its simplicity; it has many disadvantages: inevitable gastric irritation; the fact that such substances require oily or alcoholic solvents which are not well tolerated; and above all, the fact that, if intensive treatment is commenced, the patient loses his appetite completely, his mouth is constantly bad and pasty and gastric or intestinal pains sometimes develop. The disadvantages of this situation are clear, particularly in cases of serious or chronic ailments.[57]
The digestive tract should be exclusively reserved for nutrition.

4. Finally, the rectal route, used in exceptional cases. Although frequently recommended, it is not often used because it is uncomfortable and not very practical.[58]

Why not add cutaneous absorption to this list?[59]
Physiology teaches us that the skin absorbs neither water nor dissolved substances if it is healthy and intact. Nevertheless, "it is possible to make the skin absorb volatile substances at body temperature" (Arthus), a fact confirmed by Linossier's experiments. To this, Hédon adds a correction which will subsequently be taken into account: non-absorption via the skin is due to the insulating layer of sebum and, if this coating is removed, the skin then absorbs "quite actively" (Hédon).
Therefore, the absorption of volatile substances has been demonstrated physiologically and clinically and most antiseptic substances used in treating pulmonary ailments are volatile. Maximum absorption will be achieved if the product is brought to body temperature and if the sebum coating the skin is first thoroughly removed. The skin must therefore first be thoroughly cleansed with

a solvent or with the substance used, even where it is volatile.[60]

It is thus apparent that a product intended for pulmonary antisepsis administered by cutaneous absorption must fulfil two conditions:

1. It must be volatile, yet not too volatile because, when applied, too much of the liquid would dissipate into the air;[61]

2. It must dissolve fats rapidly and readily to ensure the fast and effective penetration of the active substance.

Hitherto, substances available for revulsion were intended exclusively for that purpose, with no consideration given to the "absorption" effect. Furthermore, in general, the desired goal was attained, with the revulsion achieved equal to that which would have been produced by a mustard plaster or poultice.

This therapeutic method was therefore not fully exploited; the fact that slightly irritated skin cleansed of oil is an excellent channel for absorption was left out of account.

Indeed, if eucalyptus, guaiacol or thymol, which is a perfect antiseptic,[62] is dissolved in an alcohol or ether-alcohol mixture, this will produce not only a revulsive reaction but also the rapid absorption of these various substances.

This absorption will take place via several channels:

a) Firstly directly via the skin, which has become semi-permeable, to the pleura and the lungs;

b) Via the respiratory tract as, when the substance is applied, the ambient air contains a certain amount of the product in its gaseous state. After acting on the bronchial tubes and the lungs, the product re-enters the blood and the following is created:

c) An absorption channel via the bloodstream; initially via the pulmonary alveoli and then via small vasodilated vessels in the skin, the subcutaneous cell tissue and the muscles at the point of application.

Therefore, due to the extreme diffusibility of the substance, all the pulmonary alveoli will be affected by the active substance, by the air circulating in them and by the blood irrigating them.

Some products such as guaiacol need to be used carefully

because they can cause hypothermia. It is difficult to perfect a substance of this kind as one must never forget that the revulsion effect is only sought because of the absorption effect it produces.

An established substance of this kind can be used in the following ways:

a) Firstly, as a prophylactic before and after surgery. One application should be sufficient to prevent pulmonary complications, particularly in cases of surgery on the stomach, the pleuropulmonary system or the urogenital tract:

– in ailments where pulmonary complications are particularly frequent and serious, such as coryza, tracheitis, otitis, and in infectious diseases, especially scarlet fever, mumps and measles;

– to produce a reaction in patients who are cold due to shock, drowning, serious trauma etc.

b) As a curative:

– for chronic ailments, such as pulmonary tuberculosis, cutaneous absorption of antiseptic and healing substances can only be beneficial, if for the sole reason that such substances have a gentle action on the digestive tract – an extremely important factor in such cases.

In other cases such as fetid bronchitis, bronchiectasis and pulmonary gangrene, cutaneous absorption should be used concurrently with respiratory, subcutaneous and intramuscular absorption.

– In acute ailments such a substance is definitely indicated as this method causes strong revulsion and antisepsis *loco dolenti*. Thus it can be widely used in cases of bronchitis, pneumonia, bronchopneumonia, pleural ailments, pleural and lung suppuration etc.

THE DISADVANTAGES OF FATTY SUBSTANCES

Professor Loeper, citing the skin as an absorption path, speaks of the possibility of using ointments which should be of a high titre and which therefore are not totally safe. This method, which is then in fact rejected by Professor Loeper, has no sound physiological basis. Although the ideal solution is to remove grease from the skin, should lanoline or vaseline be used as a carrier for the active substance?

Do ointments then have no redeeming features? Yes – they have one, albeit rather artificial: they help medicine penetrate the skin mechanically by repeated friction (this is what happens with the liniment used in massage; absorption is purely local. This is true of all ointments).

On the other hand, the use of specifically active volatile products, such as selected essential oils, produces a physiological, and not mechanical, absorption resulting in total diffusion rather than localised action.

No real penetration of menthol or guaiacol into the system can occur following the application of ointments based on these substances. They can only penetrate skin which has been thoroughly degreased and in which the blood vessels are dilated.[63]

The skin is a membrane which can be made temporarily permeable to volatile substances with a known action. This simple observation constitutes an original, active, reliable and harmless therapeutic method (Sassard).

Aromatic revulsion has now been successfully practised for some years with all previous theoretical data proving valid in practice.

Less violent revulsion is highly effective not only for all types of bronchial ailments, but also for most local pains, rheumatic or otherwise. It also dissipates extravasation of blood and eliminates ecchymosis (bruising) by stimulating vasodilation and thus fluidising the blood.

Revulsion using turpentine oil is an old practice which is not without its disadvantages. At certain stages of oxidation, turpentine oil can cause epidermal exfoliation and burns of varying degrees while the tiny quantity of aromatic alcohols found with pinene in this unpleasant smelling oil are not sufficiently efficacious. Mustard essence is unstable, arnica essence is not commercial. For massages,[64] Renaudet recommends arnica, calamus, mace, rue, juniper, savin, rosemary, thyme, wild thyme, lavender, yellow amber, birch and wintergreen.

Finally, let us mention the rapid absorption by the skin of vitamins and hormones, which have an undeniable action on the organism. When used with essential oils, these substances are surprisingly effective.

Narcosis Accidents and Revulsion Using Essential Oils

Narcosis[65] is achieved by means of highly volatile substances such as sulphuric ether, chloroform, ethyl chloride etc., or by a mixture of similar volatile substances.

During surgery, the patient's lungs are filled with a mixture of air and the vapours of these substances which have a very low boiling point. Once narcosis is achieved, the body temperature drops several degrees and the blood flow, thus slowed down, transports only a far lower number of calories to the tissues.

Accidents frequently result, the most feared of which is operation pneumonia.

Serious efforts have been made to determine the mechanism of this often fatal complication, the incidence of which varies regionally, affecting from three to eight per cent of operated patients, often with fatal consequences. One suspected cause is the drastic cooling of the pulmonary alveoli as a result of the production of a sort of refrigerant mixture, for, where there is a sufficient quantity of volatile substances immiscible with water, the pressure of the vapours from the ether used and water vapour combine and, due to the relative vacuum created by the movement of the ribs and the diaphragm, the evaporation generates cold by exactly the same mechanism as that used in refrigerators.

Additionally, the sluggish blood flow does not carry the heat needed and the cooled, devitalised tissues become inflamed and then contract pneumonia.

Another suspected cause is ischaemia of the blood caused when organic liquids immiscible with water saturate the alveoli and small vessels and dehydrate the tissues. The lung becomes pallid and bloodless. The resultant drop in gaseous exchanges and the lack of haemoglobin oxidation cause both the onset of asphyxia and a general fall in temperature and, as the lungs are cooled the most, they are the first to feel the effects.

Narcosis accidents can be aggravated by impurities in narcotics and by the nature of these impurities, for statistics reveal periods and regions in which accidents are more frequent than at other times or elsewhere, thus leading to the conclusion that one batch of a narcotic sold in a given region was more dangerous than another.

Nonetheless, although certain mixtures of volatile substances seem less dangerous than others, they all induce serious cooling and subsequent complications which are often fatal.

Proposed safeguards have produced mediocre or inconsistent results. Hitherto, only one has proven supreme and definitive to the point that, in the clinics, hospitals and regions where it is systematically and routinely used, there have not been ANY fatal accidents for several years. The number of lives spared in this way is considerable in the large surgical centres which use this measure.

Accidents nonetheless observed have shown that, either as a result of negligence or forgetfulness, this method was not applied. These very rare accidents therefore confirm that, where the method of essential oil revulsion is not used, accidents can occur with the same narcotics which produce no accidents if the stated precautions are systematically applied.

This method is revulsion using essential oils.[66]

Revulsion by means of poultices, a method used in some clinics, is difficult, impractical and complicated. It produces extra moisture on the cutaneous surface which is sometimes exposed to the air. When this moisture evaporates, it causes fluctuations of hot and cold which are more dangerous than the failure to take any precautionary measures.

In contrast, revulsion with essential oils leaves the skin dry and warm with revulsion continuing for the entire duration of the operation and thereafter. Vasodilation in the thoracic wall tissue is sufficiently stimulated to minimise the temperature drop in the pulmonary region and prevent congestion.

The essential oil revulsive is prepared using terpenic substances from plants. It is a white, aromatic liquid which gives a sensation of heat or even a certain degree of burning. It is applied with a large brush on the front and back of the thorax, from the shoulders down to the waist.

The sensation of heat or even burning may seem unbearable to a conscious patient but is well tolerated by the unconscious patient.

Thus, the revulsive is generously applied to each patient when brought to the operating table. Immediately after the operation, or when the patient regains consciousness, the same treatment is repeated (with a thinner layer of the revulsive if the patient is highly sensitive). It has been noted that when the patient regains consciousness, there is a reduced feeling of nausea and the patient has a particular sensation of well-being and euphoric warmth. In addition, the aromatic vapours are slowly inhaled when the patient is sleeping or awake and ensure complete antisepsis of the air passages, thus preventing any possible spread of germs.

Many patients insistently ask for additional applications of the revulsive for several days following the operation. Nuns or nurses working in wards with inadequate stocks of this revulsive have likewise been known to borrow it from neighbouring wards so as not to omit this procedure which produces such consistent and reliable results.

No accidents have been recorded for two years now in the clinics and surgical departments in the Lyon region which routinely and systematically use revulsion before surgery.

Pre- and post-operative revulsion thus seems today to be the only method which gives consistent and reliable results without any appreciable complications.

No contraindications have been reported although tens of thousands of applications have been made on patients suffering from illnesses of all kinds.

THE ACTION OF ESSENCES ON THE NERVOUS CENTRES[67]

The very nature of natural human and animal odoriferous secretions and the fact that they are produced mainly during sexual arousal, firstly brought to mind the action of perfumes on the nervous centres (*Odeurs et parfums, leur influence sur le sens génésique* [Odours and perfumes, their effect on the procreative instinct], Dr Et. Tardif, 1896). Animal scents were used throughout the ancient world, in the Orient and in Africa, as aphrodisiacs (*El Kiab, Des lois secrètes de l'amour, d'après le Khodja Omer Haleby Abou Othman* [El Kiab, The secret laws of love according to the Khodja Omer Haleby Abou Othman], translated by Paul de Regla, 1893).

However, ancient doctors were already using essences to cure hysterical or hysteriform convulsions. Treatment with fragrant vapours stopped the fits almost instantaneously.

Musk, amber and civet, says Fonssagrives, act more by their volatile and scented constituents than by their other constituents. In the past, epilepsy attacks were prevented primarily by the vapours released from heated amber; however, it is possible that the attacks halted in this way were not fits caused by epilepsy but more benign problems. Nonetheless, this information, even if it is inaccurate, is based on the realisation of the true antispasmodic value of this substance which has its maximum effect when inhaled.

Castoreum, which also enjoyed a tremendous reputation, and musk from musk deer may be more effective when inhaled than when administered either in the form of cynogloss pills, enemas of tincture of musk or "Karabé" amber syrup.

According to Francis Marre, the odours given off by heliotrope and vanilla are antispasmodic and help soothe emotional manifestations of varying degrees of gravity, commonly known as "hysterics".

Hawthorn essence (*Cratægus oxyacantha L*) is considered to be a mild cardiac. Fiessingue called it the valerian of the heart. Its sedative cardio-nervine effects influence principally the vascular system. Arterial hypertension abates after prolonged use over several months (Dr Ferrua).

Neroli essence and orangeflower water are tranquillisers which slow the heart beat substantially. F. Grégoire's experiments on isolated frogs' hearts (*Etudes physico-chimique et physiologique des eaux distillées aromatiques* [Physico-chemical and physiological studies of aromatic distilled waters], 1930) provide impressive graphs of remarkable clarity. A 2/1,000 solution of pure benzaldehyde[68] causes the heart to stop abruptly and immediately with spasms. A 2/10,000 solution stops the heart after a progressive decrease in the height of the systoles, with no spasms. Laurel waters, also containing hydrocyanic acid, stop the heart with no spasms. Methyl anthranilate[69] solutions act by slowing the heartbeat, like the action of orangeflower water.

The introduction of distilled mint water into the same frog heart causes a gradual fall in the amplitude of the systoles. Rosewater either causes the heart to stop after a slow and gradual reduction in the amplitude of the contractions, or causes an abrupt halt with no prior decrease in systolic height.

Essence of melissa is considered to be an antispasmodic and valerian essence a tranquilliser. Dr M. P. Marceval says that the essences of clove, sage, myrtle and rose stimulate the sexual centres with no functional disturbance, whereas others such as camphor, asafoetida and calamus essences and camphorated oils act in the opposite way.

Mr Léopold Gache, a pharmacist, has, for his part, studied a certain number of hypnotic[70] essences but has not made a list of them.

Cajeput essence is antineuralgic and antihysteric.

Angelica essence, at low doses, stimulates the brain, but at high doses it becomes a narcotic. Japanese (ketonic) camphor is a sedative. Borneol (camphor of Borneo) is a stimulant. Almost all essential oils are analgesic.[71]

Cadéac and Meunier state that savory essence is a stimulant and narcotic. A low dose is sufficient to modify innervation and motivity significantly. A dose of 30 drops of savory essence, taken on an empty stomach, initially produces a general numbness with a marked sensation of cold. After half an hour, the head clears, mental activity is stimulated and intellectual work becomes easier. A feeling of well-being and of strength results. This second phase lasts several hours.

At therapeutic doses, savory essence is always a tonic for the heart. At toxic doses, two periods are observed, the first characterised by an increase in the number and the strength of heartbeats and by a significant drop in arterial tension and the second by a gradual weakening of the pulse (A. Sassard).

Mental predispositions sometimes considerably reinforce the effect of essential oils and thus experimentation is not always easy, except on animals.[72] Toxic reactions can sometimes be produced simply by autosuggestion. Nevertheless, the comments made by Mr G. Guislain and Guy Laroche can be considered accurate when they state that certain essences increase neurosis and can cause epileptic fits. To observe this action, they intoxicated rabbits with essential oil of tansy. The central nervous systems of these animals were crushed without the addition of any excipient. When injected at a dose of 0.2 cm³ into a guinea pig's dura mater, it caused convulsions and a fatal coma within eight to ten hours. While the dose of tansy essence injected into the rabbit was not fatal but only caused convulsions, the rabbit's medulla oblongata alone is toxic to the guinea pig. These experiments seem to demonstrate the selective action of essences on the central nervous system and in particular on the area of the bulb. Tansy essence is rich in thujone (ketone) and thus one of the most toxic known.[73]

We will see in the chapter on the toxicity of essential oils that, with a few exceptions (especially ketonic essences), essential oils constitute a danger to the nervous system only at high doses, where their elimination, albeit very rapid and very intensive via the respiratory and renal systems, is not fast enough.

ACTION ON THE DIGESTIVE TRACT

Essences are sialagogic (that is, they encourage saliva secretion, the first stage in digestion), and this is why the use of masticatories (used for thousands of years in the Far East) is so widespread in America and even in Europe, with betel, mastic, catechu and flavoured chewing gum consumed in large quantities.

Aromatic sweets and liqueurs are eupeptic[74] and, when taken in moderate amounts, are only beneficial to the digestion. Spices and aromatic seasonings, widely used in hot countries, act in two ways. Firstly, they are anti-putrefactive and prevent food from rotting too quickly and, secondly, they stimulate all the digestive functions. The quantity of seasonings used throughout the world far exceeds that of essential oils (on the basis of aromatic value) used for all other known applications.

It can be said that aromatic diets are the norm around the world and that the amount of aromatic substances humans absorb goes far beyond anything we would imagine (see Spices and Condiments, by Stanley Redgrove, London, 1933).

The most well-known effect of essential oils on the intestines consists of the expulsion of gas which causes borborygmi.[75] Caraway, fennel and aniseed are the main oils used for this purpose. This action can be explained by the activation of peristalsis movements (Georges Renaudet). If certain essences are introduced into the intestines in keratin capsules, secretion is intensified, digestion accelerated and sometimes there is even slight purging by exosmosis. Essences are cholagogue[76] and laxative. Antiseptic by nature, they also have the virtue of disinfecting the digestive organs (Dr Forgues).

Rosemary essence is a stomachic medicine, beneficial in treating atonic dyspepsia. It is a stimulant and a tonic (Dr Brissemoret, *Essai sur les préparations galéniques* [Essay on galenical preparations]).

The kidneys react differently to different essences, although almost all essences are diuretics. The diuretic properties of juniper berries, common lovage and angelica root and parsley have always been known and have been attributed to the essences of these plants. Balsamic plants such as sandalwood, cedar, copaiba etc. are also diuretics.

Dr Faulds' observations on the use of eucalyptus leaf infusions for treating *diabetes mellitus* do not seem to be necessarily attributed to the essential oil.

Our experiments on the decrease in alcoholic symptoms when

aromatic alcohols are ingested demonstrated to us the considerable diuretic effect of most essential oils on guinea pigs. When examined in autopsy, the guinea pig's kidneys were still healthy except where ketonic essences were used.

Dr Forgues states that phenolic essences of thyme and oregano also irritate the kidneys and give rise to constant diuresis.

Professor B. Cabasse has cited the interesting property of several aromatic gums of preventing the formation of certain types of ulcers of the digestive tract, caused by tobacco or alcohol abuse.

Too many strong drinks taken between meals can cause stomach cancer in subjects who were otherwise not predisposed to this almost incurable disease.

Smoker's cancer is also due to immoderate tobacco abuse, although there are also other determining factors. All smokers are potential victims of irritation or even ulcerated lesions of the mucous membranes of the mouth and pharynx which can provoke the onset of this terrible disease.

Smoker's cancer is practically unknown in the Levant, the home of the finest tobaccos, and Professor Cabassè thus sought the reason for this and found it in the Orientals' habit of chewing a resin called olibanum or frankincense. This resinous gum of the boswellia family originated in India and is an ingredient of a large number of masticatory mixtures. It has a pleasant balsamic smell, a slightly bitter taste, and softens when chewed. It was a precious ingredient of the incense used for religious purposes where it was used, according to Malmonides, to mask the smell of the blood of sacrificed animals, but Arabic doctors also used it as a remedy, even for cancer.

Recent works by Italian doctors state that essences minimise the toxic effects of tobacco. It should be added that, according to Cabassè's work, they also reduce the irritation to the mucous membranes and heal them before they became dangerous.[77]

As terpenes are always irritants of the digestive organs,[78] we would recommend the use of terpeneless essential oils whenever possible.

THE ACTION OF ESSENCES
ON THE SKIN

From time immemorial, essences have been used to treat skin diseases. However, whether these products truly have a greater effect or whether ancient medicine was more familiar with "aromatic infused oils"[79] than with steam-distilled essences, we must recognize that doctors in ancient times mostly used what today is called "oil of cade". This oil was not only the tar of *Juniperus oxycedrus* but also that of the cedar. This was established beyond doubt by the pharmacist, Commander M. Massy, in his study entitled *Le cèdre de l'Atlas et les produits qu'il fournit à la thérapeutique* [The Atlas cedar and the products it provides for therapeutic uses].

The cedria of Pliny or Dioscorides is in fact the tar from the cedar of Lebanon and it is still used everywhere this magnificent tree grows. Buchoz, in his Dissertation, in 1806, on the cedar of Lebanon, mentions cedar oil which is so strongly recommended for treating scabies and skin sores.

Tested by Dr Lépinay (at the Casablanca clinic) for the treatment of psoriasis, dandruff, ringworm and, generally, all skin conditions for which oil of cade is indicated, empyreumatic *Cedrus atlantica* oil has always proven to be at least as good as true oil of cade.

The doctors Decrop and Salle, in Fez, and Dr Noiré have the same favourable view of this substance as the ancients did of cedria. It can be used in the form of glycerols, ointments, cerates and emulsions or it can be brushed on in its pure state. R. Huerre (*Bulletin Génerale de Thérapeutique* [General Journal of Therapeutics], 1914) states moreover that empyreumatic products can be replaced to good effect by steam-distilled essential oils (for treating pityriasis, dandruff, seborrhoea, traumatic alopecia, psoriasis, patchy alopecia etc.).

It is clear that many essential oils other than wood oils (cade or cedar) give identical results.

Balsam of Peru has long been used for these same diseases. Dr Peter, of Prague, invented the method and imported it to Paris where he put it into practice, in particular at St. Lazare. In 1896, M. Descouleurs wrote his doctoral thesis on this subject and did comparative tests of balsams on lice. Dr Julien, for his part, made many observations on the same subject, but balsam of Peru, like tar, is resinous as well as aromatic and acts against scabies both mechanically and chemically. We have been able to demonstrate that all essential oils, in particular those from labiate plants,[80] when dissolved either in fatty oils or in Turkey red oil soaps produce the same result much more simply as these mixtures are removed just by rinsing with warm water, unlike plasters of balsam of Peru, tar, cade or cedar.

All forms of pityriasis[81] can be cured in this way.

Essence of thuja is used by a Polish doctor to treat warts and persistent condylomas either by brushing it on the affected area or by injecting it close to the warts. As a result of this treatment, the warts dry out and fall off after a lukewarm bath.

According to Dr Annie Bailey of Dambury, Connecticut, essence of hyssop is an excellent remedy for all skin diseases caused by defective blood composition, such as leprosy, syphilitic sores – especially in the tertiary stage – scrofula, cancerous growths and various types of eczema. Dr Bailey has patients take two to three drops of essence of hyssop per day and also recommends that they drink a lot of water. However, it is preferable to stop all other medication (quoted by A. Sassard).

The irritant action of certain essential oils, in the form of ointments, is rarely used these days. Only compound rosemary ointment (*Unguentum nervinum*) is still used to a certain extent. In addition to rosemary, it contains the essential oil of bay and juniper oil (*Pharmacopoeia boruscica*).

The nerve balsam in the *Codex medicamentarius gallicus* contains, among other substances, nutmeg butter and essence of cloves which gives it its Latinised name of *Pomatum muscitae compositum*. Lebas' veterinary nerve ointment contains sage, lavender, rosemary and thyme.

Solutions of essences obtained either by direct solubility in water or dispersion in soap also produce very good results. In the form of creamy acid pH emulsions, some essential oils produce interesting results when used on all types of skin irritations in children or on scalp irritations in adults, as a supplement to aromatic solutions for treating all types of dermatosis, pruritus, bedsores, cracks in the skin, chapping etc. (Dr P. Sassard).

DR MEURISSE'S OBSERVATIONS

Chronic perianal and perineal eczema. Sixty-year-old neuroarthritic woman with a tendency to obesity. Eczema first appeared two years ago, around the anus, on the perineum and the labia majora: acute, weeping, highly pruriginous[82] eczema. Lesions became chronic, intense itching, especially at night, despite repeated applications of St. Louis formula ointment.

Upon examination: chronic eczema, lesions from scratching and areas of lichenification. Treatment commenced on 15th May after a bout of influenza with congestion of the right lung and a slight uraemic crisis; treatment ended on 12th June. Daily application of terpeneless lavender oil, then, after a few minutes, powdered with talc and bismuth. At bedtime: camphorated, sulphurated cade balsam. Pruritus quickly abated, lesions receded, the areas of lichenification abated and left in their stead pigmented patches. The improvement was very rapid and the day the patient left us, the eczema, which had resisted treatment for two years, had almost disappeared.

DR MARCHAND'S OBSERVATIONS

The Scalp

Mrs X, 28 years old, losing large quantities of hair; pityriasis[83] despite constant care, use of lotions, scalp massage, shampoos etc.; considerable hair loss and, as usual, particularly around the parietal and occipital bones. Unbearable itching, insomnia, head-aches, heavy-headed feeling. In my presence, a large quantity of hair came away at a slight tug. The scalp was dry, covered with dandruff. First application of pure terpeneless lavender oil on small cottonwool balls held by tweezers. Massage between small sections of hairs.

On 29th April, the patient returned very satisfied. Delighted, she emphasized the following points: the massage had none of the disadvantages of an ointment; she did it rather late in the afternoon and it did not stain her pillow as she wore a small cap.

Today her hair is shiny, beautiful, light and full of body. The itching has stopped completely. Her nights are undisturbed. Observations about appearance: the wave done yesterday before the consultation has not changed. The scalp is almost free of dandruff. Hair colour has not changed.

Second application by the same method. On 1st May, some hair fell out again. Scalp itself is shiny, clean.

F. Soldier, Fourth Engineers. Case of alopecia with numerous large patches. Daily use of pure lavender lotions; cured rapidly.

Venereology

Essences and balsams have consistently been used for the treatment of diseases of the urinary tract. Commenting on this use, Georges Renaudet says that, while not a specific remedy, essences disinfect urine and prevent the development of gonococci.[84] The Technical Section of the Military Health Department also stated that essence of Atlas cedar (cedar of Lebanon, *Cedrus atlantica*) acts on the pain factor and the duration of flow. Many essences are anti-gonorrheic. Cubeb essence, *Dipterocarpus turbinatus* Gaernt. essence from *D. alatus* Roxb. and the various types of gurjun balsam are mentioned in addition to sandalwood essence and copaiba balsam (John Maisch, A Manual of Organic Materia Medica, 1890; and Henry Kraemer, A Textbook of Botany and Pharmacognosy, 1910). Matico[85] essence reportedly has the same merits.

A special place must be given to the essence of *Cedrus atlantica*, firstly because it is a home-produced substance, which Moroccan production can expand if need be and, at least on the French market, take the place of Indian or Australian products.

Professor Trabut pioneered the therapeutic use of essence of Atlas cedar. In 1899, at Mustapha hospital in Algiers, Professor Gemy conducted certain experiments and concluded from them that African Cedar essence is second to none and that it has the advantage of having no adverse effect on the digestive tract or the kidneys. Dosages vary from author to author: Dr Raynaud prescribes 1.6 grams per day, Dr Huertas increases the dose initially to 6 and 7 grams. The chief physician, Dr Bichelonne, prescribes 2 grams initially, increasing to 8 grams and then gradually decreasing the dosage. More recent experiments by Drs Evrard, Tant, Duffaut and Jausion (professor of medicine at Val de Grâce Hospital) confirm these statements. Cedar essence, like many others, is also said to be effective against rheumatic pains, atonic wounds (Huertas) and all manner of other diseases when used in potions, inhalants, throat washes, ointments etc. (Boisse). It has not yet been possible to determine the extent to which sesquiterpenic alcohols, cadinene (sesquiterpene) or other constituents act as therapeutic agents. Although it contains far less sesquiterpenic alcohol than sandalwood essence, *Cedrus atlantica* essence produces the same results at the same dosages. Copaiba balsam, which contains no alcohols, is also very effective (Pharmacist Commander M. Massy, 1928, *Le Cèdre de l'Atlas et les produits qu'il fournit à la thérapeutique* [The Atlas cedar and the products it provides for therapeutic uses]).

Thus, essences have a fairly general action and, indeed, the trials we conducted with Dr J. Marchand of Lyon show that lavender essence acts in the same way as the above-mentioned essences, in keratin capsules and at relatively low doses (1 to 2 grams per day). Lavender essence also acts remarkably well in the healing of venereal sores such as chancroids[A], cankerous adenitis,[B] phagedenas[C] and syphilitic gummas.[D] The observations below define the conditions of use of this essence.

DR MARCHAND'S OBSERVATIONS[86]

D.M. 113th R.A., admitted on 7th April, 1918. Diagnosis: soft chancroid in groove. First treated with wet dressings until bacteriological examination revealed *Haemophilus ducreyi*. 10th April, first application of lavender essence, aristol powder, dry dressing. 14th April, very noticeable improvement. 24th April, patient left healed.

V. Maurius, 14th Service Corps. Admitted on 23rd March, 1918. Diagnosis: soft chancroid in groove. Haemophilus ducreyi present. The sore, which initially improved under the standard treatment (zinc chloride, iodoform), remained stationary, as in the previous case. 11th April, first application of lavender essence. Same treatment on subsequent days. 26th April, patient left, healed.

R. of the Italian infantry. Soft chancroid on the prepuce, *Haemophilus ducreyi*. Same treatment, same result. An attack of adenitis on the left side during this time was reabsorbed under the effect of tincture of iodine.

C. 44th R.I., admitted on 10th March. Soft chancroid on the prepuce, left inguinal adenitis. Normal treatment ineffective. On 11th April, first application of lavender essence. Perfectly healed by 25th.

M. 3rd Rifles. Admitted on 12th March. Soft chancroid on the prepuce; normal treatment had left an atonic sore. 21st April, first application of lavender essence. By 25th April, the sore had closed and, by 3rd May, it had healed completely.

R.A. Rifles. Admitted on 21st March. Soft chancroids on the prepuce and the sheath. *Haemophilus ducreyi*. Following traditional treatment, the chancroids appeared to have reached the state of stationary sclerosis already mentioned in the other cases. 21st April, first application of lavender. 22nd April, the sore was clean and pink; immediate improvement. 2nd May, almost completely healed. 7th May, patient left, healed.

D. Jules 152nd R.I., admitted on 20th May. Soft chancroid on the prepuce, balanitis.[E] *Haemophilus ducreyi*, no treponemas. Treated immediately with lavender essence. Good progress by 31st May. Left, healed, on 6th June.

G. Marcel, 4th Engineers, admitted on 1st May. Wide syphilitic chancre (size of a two-franc coin) on the prepuce. The sore was healing slowly with silver nitrate and calomel ointment; the mercurial treatment had been applied from the first day. On 11th May, we decided to try lavender essence. By 22nd May, the chancre was half healed, the sore was closing very quickly and by 29th was completely healed.

Ch. F. 5th Rifles. Admitted on 25th March. Syphilitic chancre on the fraenum, the anal groove and the prepuce. Wet dressings the first few days. Presence of *Treponemas*[F] on 10th; lavender essence on 11th; completely healed on 24th.

Jean C. Third C.M. Two superficial leg wounds. Application on 24th and 25th July. Healed on 26th.

C. 413th R.I., sore on left arm. Healed in three days.

W. Tsi-To, colonial worker. Chancroid on the prepuce. Impossible to specify origin and date (*Haemophilus ducreyi*). Admitted on 4th March, left, healed, on 19th.

V.G., admitted on 4th March. Multiple soft chancroids on the prepuce, clearly raised ulcerations; seven granulating. *Haemophilus ducreyi*. Improvement on 6th March: all but two lesions had flattened; they looked like pinkish erosions bleeding slightly; very little suppuration. All the ulcerations had flattened by 12th. Patient discharged, healed, on 19th March.

P. Soft chancroid on the prepuce, dating back 15 days; admitted on 26th January, 1919. Almost healed by 5th February. Left, healed, on 12th.

V. Two soft chancroids located in the anal groove. Numerous *Haemophilus ducreyi*, polynucleic, various cocci. Quickly healed. Returned on 4th March with suppurated adenitis on right. Incision on 5th March. Healed and discharged on 20th March.

P.P. Gendarme, admitted on 4th January. Suppurating left inguinal adenitis. Soft chancroid on the prepuce not healed; this chancre required a 51-day stay in hospital at Amiens, 20 intramuscular and six intravenous injections.

Incision of the bubo, injection of lavender into the empty bubo followed by dressing with lavender. Left for the front on 21st January.

M.B., 27th March. Syphilis at the age of 16 years. Positive Wassermann test at the Pasteur Institute in 1917. Tertiary lesion of the fourth toe on the left foot. Shallow, infected, suppurating lesion. The sore was almost totally healed by the third application. Mercurial treatment every other day. Healed by the 10th day. This patient had been trying all manner of products for a period of four months: calomel ointments etc.

DR MEURISSE'S OBSERVATIONS

Young man, 19 years old, with mild case of gonorrhoea. Some discharge; pus globules with intracellular gonococci present. Discharge stopped in 12 days after washes with terpeneless lavender with 1% Turkey red oil.[G] Gonococci disappeared by the tenth day. Beer test on the 25th day, discharge did not reappear.

Twenty-seven-year-old man with acute blennorrhoea.[87] Heavy greenish discharge; erections and urination painful, numerous gonococci. Rest, emollient drinks, internal urotropin daily baths, 0.10 camphor bromate, three to four pills per night. Whole-body washes at slight pressure with 5 per thousand solution Salvone (solution of labiate essences and Turkey red oil), twice a day. Rapid decrease of discharge in eight days, urination no longer painful, slight yellowish discharge, erections no longer painful, some gonococci still present. On the thirteenth day, as Salvol injection was becoming painful, washing with 5/1,000 solution of lavender essence in water boiled with linseed. No more gonococci by the twentieth day. Healed by the twenty-seventh day.

Blennorrhagic vaginitis in eight-year-old girl, origin unknown; father and mother have no gonococci. The child was very tired, had rings under her eyes; the vulva was inflamed, covered with a greenish, foul-smelling pus; subfebrile state, tongue slightly coated.
    Rest, milk, emollient herbal teas, urotropin; vaginal injections twice daily with 5/1,000 Salvol in boiled water; after two days, injections with 10/1,000 Salvol in boiled water.
    20th May, numerous pus globules, pavement cells, some isolated, some in thick patches, numerous intracellular gonococci. 22nd May, lessening of discharge, fewer gonococci, some intact polynuclears and some mononuclears. 24th May, the pus is more liquid, epithelial debris; some gonococci every third field.
    Application of a lavender essence bougie.[88]
    2nd June: no gonococci.
    12th June: healed definitively, monitored thereafter.

DR FORGUES' OBSERVATIONS

Phagedenic chancre around the penis. Fifteen-minute applications of strong solution in compresses (30 grams per litre of a 20% solution of Turkey red oil in water, i.e. six grams lavender essence per litre of water) for two weeks; unexpectedly *restitutio ad integrum*.

Syphilitic gumma in the nasal fossae. Mercurial treatment did not produce the expected results at all: the sore remained open and sanious. Permanent dressings of a weak solution (three grams of essence per litre of water) produced the following two results of prime importance: elimination of the purulent discharge with deodorisation and opening of the nasal fossae after 14 days.

OBSTETRICS AND GYNAECOLOGY

After having had trials conducted in 1916 at the hospital of Padua, we asked Dr Meurisse to carry out a certain number of experiments which were summarised at the time in the brochure entitled *La thérapeutique par les huiles essentielles* [Therapy with Essential Oils[89]] (1919, Dr Paul Meurisse, former head of the Bacteriology Laboratory of the fifteenth region).

"Uterine and utero-salpingo-ovarian ailments", he says, "are often stubborn and expose the 'afflicted' to such hopelessly long treatments that the poor women sometimes ask the surgeon for the merciful operation to rid them of their diseased organs or, weary of so much vain treatment, abandon therapy altogether. We have tried every method and can state that failures are often due to the inadequacy of the means employed. We are therefore now convinced that Salvol (a water-miscible mixture of essences) has major benefits either as a therapeutic method in the hands of a doctor caring for a patient, or for hygiene purposes as no other antiseptic is so pleasant to use. It can be recommended as effective in personal hygiene, douches, sitz baths and full baths. Applications on the cervix, vaginal and intra-uterine douches, glycerol-coated tampons, all using essences, have in all cases produced the desired cures" (Dr Meurisse).

Since that time, we have created new essence-based preparations with new saponaceous excipients for better dispersion of the volatile elements.

We have used new mixtures of essential oils and constituents and have studied the effects of the pH of the solutions thus obtained. With the help of Dr Sassard, mentioned on many occasions in this work, we have been able to develop other products, with even more consistent results than those produced by Salvol, with labiate essences.

In all cases of metritis[90] and cervicitis,[91] the aromatic solution rapidly sedates all the phenomena of inflammation and the weeping, ulcerated or fungous cervices regain their colour and normal consistency and heal. In obstetrics, *ante and post partum* aromatic baths are one of the best preventive measures against all forms of puerperal infection. Vaginal douches, pessaries inserted at night and followed by a douche transform even the most diseased cervices after just a few applications and at the same time rapidly reduce inflammation throughout the entire pelvis minor.

DR MEURISSE'S OBSERVATIONS (GYNAECOLOGY)

Observation. Twenty-four-year-old woman, metritis of the cervix following a miscarriage at two months. Heavy whitish-yellowish discharge staining underwear; heaviness of the lower abdomen when walking or fatigued; constipation; frequent desire to urinate. Slight prolapse of the uterus, body resistant to pressure on the cervix. Examination with a speculum revealed slightly enlarged cervix, labia minora granulate with slight discharge.

Treatment: Salvol applied to the cervix; vaginal injections with 15 grams per two litres of water, tampons with glycerised Salvol. Treatment continued three times per week for two and a half months. At this time, slight irregular discharge of colourless mucus; the size of the lower part of the uterus had greatly decreased and the *os uteri externum* had regained its normal colour. No pain when walking.

Thirty-five-year-old woman has had three pregnancies without incident. At end of May, miscarriage at two and a half months, apparently caused by a fall. Severe haemorrhaging began a few days after the fall. Ejection of foetus, induced labour. The placenta gave off a slight odour. Warm injections of 10/1,000 Salvol. Lochia[92] with slight unpleasant smell during the first three days, followed by light draining with a gauze dressing soaked in 20% Salvol.

Thirty-seven-year-old woman. Two previous pregnancies; the last one, six years ago, ended with a forceps delivery. Following that delivery, heavy yellowish discharge, treated by a midwife then by a specialist. Unpleasant pruritis, feeling of heaviness. Slight retroversion of the uterus, cervix wide and enlarged; in short, prior metritis with slight parametritis. Intra-uterine injections with 10% Salvol glycerine; injections and glycerised tampons with the same essence. Warm baths with Salies de Béarn salts. Rest. Periods became less painful after three weeks of treatment. The second month, we also used applications of small bougies of cocoa butter and terpeneless lavender twice a week. Sitz baths with Salvol eliminated the vulvular pruritis. Improvement continued during the month of June: we applied the bougies only once a week. The great improvement was certainly due to the slow and continuous action of the lavender essence on a chronically congested and permanently discharging mucous membrane.

Thirty-three-year-old woman. Globular uterine fibroma developed principally near the left uterine cornu. Previous catarrhal endometriosis with abundant white viscous discharge with unpleasant smell, especially after periods, which are heavy and in which clots are expelled. The fibroma dated back five years. General state of health fairly good. Treatment: series of baths with Salies de Béarn salts at home, daily injections of 10/1,000 Salvol; glycerised Salvol tampons every night. Treated regularly from 10th March to 3rd May: vaginal discharge, which soon became fluid, disappeared fairly soon. Patient seen again in June and July: great improvement, no more discharge between periods which almost returned to normal; the Salies de Béarn salts reduced the size of the fibroma; patient continuing Salvol injections as she was so pleased with them.

(OBSTETRICS)

Primiparous[93] woman, 18 years old. Labour had been very difficult. Slow dilation, very long delivery which should have been shortened by use of forceps. The baby presented apparently dead and artificial respiration was necessary. Also, the meconium had been partly discharged into the uterine cavity. Labour ended in the morning of 21st March. Temp. that evening, 38.9 degrees; on the morning of the 22nd, 38.8 degrees, no albumin in urine. Temp. in evening, 40.3 degrees, foetid and malodorous lochia. Following morning, temp. 39.2 degrees; general condition unsatisfactory. We were called and prescribed two intra-uterine injections of Salvol, five grams per litre, administered slowly. Washing twice daily, Pyramidon in small doses.

By 24th, the smell of the lochia had already abated somewhat and the temperature had fallen; no smell from lochia by 25th; only one injection on 26th.

By 27th, lochia smelt normal; stopped intra-uterine injections and continued two vaginal injections per day. Healed by 15th April.

In other cases, using only intra-uterine injections, immediate powerful disinfection and deodorisation has been achieved (Dr Meurisse).

VETERINARY MEDICINE

In veterinary medicine, we obtain excellent results with mixtures of selected essences. Products containing phenols, such as thymol and eugenol, sometimes produce painful contractions: to the touch, the membranes are hard, like stretched rubber, and tighten around the hand. However, with other products such as pine oil, which is miscible with water, the membranes relax completely; they feel elastic and supple to the fist. The animals ruminate which indicates a total absence of pain.

There is therefore good reason to study special compositions of the most anaesthetic and calmative essences for intra-uterine or intravesical injections and to use essential oils which trigger contractions only where such reactions can be helpful.

Almost all essential oils are disinfectant, deodorant and healing and all can be used beneficially in normal cases. However, when movements, contractions and the tension of mucous membranes and organs need to be carefully watched and when it is desirable to prevent any pain, there is good reason to be discriminating in the choice of aromatic constituents to be used.

SOME OTHER APPLICATIONS OF ESSENCES

INFLUENZA EPIDEMIC OF 1918

In 1918, to fight influenza, we prepared a composition based on essences containing borneol and, in particular, sage essence. This composition of essences, dissolved in Turkey red oil soap, provides a stable emulsion with water (Salvol).

Since the influenza – called Spanish flu – was developing into a serious epidemic, volatile antiseptics were indicated, for it is acknowledged that influenza is transmitted primarily via the respiratory tract and the natural orifices: ears, nose, eyes, mouth. Preventive treatment consisted of gargles and nose, eye and ear drops, as long practised in hospitals housing contagious patients.

The gargles consisted of emulsions containing 6 parts per thousand of an essential oil, a dose which has a clear and rapid sterilising effect.

For the nose and ear drops, we used oil containing the same dose of essence or even the aqueous mixture above. Patients' eyes were rinsed with a 2/1,000 solution of essence which is less painful.

This treatment combined with the absorption of quinine proved to be preventive and curative (Dr Forgues). Inhalations with the same substance placed in boiling water were also often used.

AMOEBIC DYSENTERY

In treating amoebic dysentery, we replaced the traditional silver salt washes by aromatic washes with a 12 per thousand essence content, with these warm intestinal washes to be continued. The characteristic intestinal pains and the elimination of gangrenous debris ceased.

HAEMORRHOIDS

An oily cream in the acid pH range, very aromatic due to the use of terpeneless essences, in particular lavender, bergamot and geranium, immediately relieves the pruritis and the worst itching. Haemorrhoidal congestion is instantly soothed by massaging the affected areas with this cream or with a soapy solution of the same essences (Sapolinol).

CANCER

For cancer of the liver, the administration of 5 drops of hyssop essence mixed with olive oil 3 times a day is recommended (A. Sassard, pharmacist).

PLAGUE

The same mixture was used, primarily as a prophylactic agent. In a hospital for patients with the plague, all junior personnel and patients without pulmonary conditions were obliged to gargle twice a day with a 6/1,000 solution of essences and to administer nose drops of aromatic oil.

Of a staff of 35 men, over a period of 5 months, only two fatigue-men, responsible for interment, died of foudroyant[H] pneumonic plague (Dr Forgues).

The "Four Thieves Vinegar", greatly used in centuries past, was more a prophylactic than a remedy for this disease, which progresses so quickly that no attempt was even made to treat its victims.

About ten years ago, Professor Boinet of Marseille, a correspondent member of the Academy of Medicine, presented a paper about this celebrated remedy to that learned assembly.

During the plague of 1720–21, he said, it was frequently used in Marseille to fight the disease. The formula had allegedly been developed by four thieves who robbed the bodies of plague victims, without fear of the disease. When arrested, their lives were spared on condition that they divulge their formula which was immediately disclosed and posted on the walls of the city by the aldermen.

The museum of Old Marseille still has a copy of this poster. The formula was as follows:

"Take three pints of strong white wine vinegar, add a handful each of wormwood, meadowsweet, wild marjoram and sage, fifty cloves, two ounces of campanula roots, two ounces of angelica, rosemary and horehound and three large measures of camphor. Place the mixture in a container for fifteen days, strain and express, then bottle."

"Use by rubbing it on the hands, ears and temples from time to time when approaching a plague victim."

The odour of the Marseille Vinegar kept away insects and probably fleas which are known to play an important role in the propagation of this disease. The 1758 Codex modified this formula, adding rue, garlic and calamus.

It appears that the anecdote of the four thieves of Marseille is only a repetition of a much older story. The version which is probably the original is reported, according to M. A. Rolet, by a 15th century author from Auvergne as follows:

"During the former great plague (1413), four thieves went to plague victims, strangled them in their beds and then robbed their homes, for which they were condemned to be burned alive but, to lighten their sentence, they disclosed their secret protection and were hanged instead."

The people of Marseille claimed to be more lenient and grateful since they spared the lives of the four thieves. In any case and whatever its origin, this vinegar was a type of antiseptic based on aromatic substances. All modern aromatic substances using plant essences come from the Four Thieves' Vinegar, but are infinitely stronger.

EMBALMING

The embalming of corpses dates back, not to Egyptian civilization, although the practice was perfected by the Eygptians, but to earlier civilizations. It was most likely a fairly generalised practice, in the Copper Age or at the beginning of the Bronze Age, among certain peoples who, for religious reasons, abandoned the practice of cremation. The preservation of bodies became a religious rite which could not develop until the technique of preservation was adequately reliable. Mummies are found not only among the Egyptians but also among the Guanches, the Incas in America etc.*

The basis of embalming was treatment with aromatics. The nature of the balsams and essences used varied according to regional resources. Dr Reutter of Rosement endeavoured to identify the balsamics used in Egypt by analysis, despite their high degree of oxidation. In addition to natron and asphalt which constituted the basis of the process, he found turpentine, incense, mastic, styrax, the resin or tar of Atlas cedarwood and gurjun balsam.

In *Preservative materials used by the ancient Egyptian in embalming* (Cairo, 1911), Lucas gives similar information.

Dr Vidal has pointed out that this practice clearly and tangibly demonstrates the antiseptic strength of perfumes. The entire undefined flora of microbes – he states – which, immediately after death, invades a body and decomposes it, is immediately paralysed, rendered powerless and probably destroyed.

Putting our observations on the bactericidal power of lavender essence into practice, Dr Battandier, of Viriville, has been preserving bodies since 1911 with injections of thyme and lavender essence (approximately two litres per body).

Since it has now been shown that certain essential oils are harmless to living bodies, it seems obvious to deduce from this that embalming living beings is possible under certain conditions and that it should be possible to arrest certain types of septicaemias which hitherto have been considered intractable.

Non-terpenic essential oils, used in subcutaneous or intramuscular injections, are usually easily reabsorbed and, where administered

---

* The Guanches and the Incas primarily used *Chenopodium ambrosioïde* (J. Gattefossé).

in small quantities, this takes place in a matter of minutes. Injections of a mixture of terpeneless lavender and geranium essences in small animals (guinea pigs) and in the proportion of 0.5 grams per kilogram do nevertheless cause fixation abscesses (R. Cuche). However, the very mechanism of the abscess caused by turpentine oil is not itself entirely understood and it is possible that, in addition to the quantity of essential oil which becomes "fixed" locally, a certain amount diffuses little by little throughout the organism and acts as an antiseptic. Where a local abscess does not form, the essence is immediately diffused throughout the organism; the fixation of terpenes on the medulla and meningitis symptoms are observed. By creating local abscesses with essences other than turpentine and which are less rich or very low in terpenes and by avoiding essences known to act rapidly on the nervous system, it may be possible to create more effective abscesses or generalised action.

We carry out intramuscular injections on young pigs with infectious pneumonia. If the disease is caught in time, before the organs are too extensively ulcerated, rapid improvement and unexpected cures can be obtained. No abscesses have formed when we have used terpeneless Siberian pine essence, rich in borneol and bornyl acetate, at doses of 2–3 cc per day, per animal.

The external application of small quantities of essences rapidly stops the spread of gangrenous sores. In my personal experience, after a laboratory explosion covered me with burning substances which I extinguished by rolling on a grassy lawn, both my hands were covered with a rapidly developing gas gangrene. Just one rinse with lavender essence stopped "the gasification of the tissue". This treatment was followed by profuse sweating and healing began the next day (July 1910).[94]

It does therefore seem that we can expect some activity from essential oils where the practitioner seems at a loss; as for burns or injuries, the cause is well understood.

THE EMBALMING OF SORES

The surgeon Mencière used this expression at the medico-surgical meeting of the Sixth army in 1915. He advocated a method based on the use of essential oils and summarised it in the following options, each of which is for a particular stage in the development of a sore:

a) emulsion of essential oils and the principles of his balsam in water; this can be used for a wet dressing;

b) etherised solution at ten per thousand, applicable above all where large quantities of matter have been lost;

c) fatty dressings using vaseline as an excipient.

We should also note that Mencière often preceded embalming by intense phenolation which he believed would destroy as many bacterial elements as possible. The active principles of his balsam were guaiacol and eucalyptol.

In 1917, G. Duchène, for his part, recommended a formula based on vaseline and ether oil, to which he added camphor, petroleum jelly and Peru balsam.

Work carried out since the war has shown:

1. that phenolation is superfluous as essences generally have a greater bactericidal power than that of phenol and phenol has a harmful necrosing effect on tissue, contrary to essential oils which are cytophylactic;

2. that eucalyptol as a pure constituent (internal oxide or ether oxide) is not very effective and acts almost only as an excipient;

3. that guaiacol, like phenol, is caustic and is no more active than other less irritant aromatic phenols and many non-phenolic essential oils;

4. that fatty dressing are not as effective as well-aerated dressings which allow air to reach the areas which are healing;

5. with regard to Duchène's formulae: that ketonic camphor is probably less indicated than borneol (or camphor of Borneo – alcohol) and finally, that balsams, in view of their high resin content, soil the wounds and make them difficult to clean.

Despite these reservations, embalming works and, in many instances, surgery has been avoided, limbs have been saved and horrific dirty wounds have healed perfectly thanks to this method.

Since the war, some progress has been made, although the method is still not as widespread as we would like.

At the top of the list, we must cite the study of the dispersion of essential oils in liquids, the salt content of which affects cell permeability and the pH of which must be appropriate for the intended use.

The concept of antisepsis properly speaking – that is, the destruction of bacteria or the halting of their development – has lost some of its interest since it has been noted that highly-dilute solutions of essences, with an antiseptic power, proven "in vitro", apparently of zero, have excellent and extremely rapid effects.[95]

The numerous trials conducted in the hospitals of Lyon on dilute solutions of a soapy mixture containing selected essential constituents (Sapolinol), show that relatively small amounts of essential oils are required to obtain effects comparable to those achieved by Dr Forgues, Dr Meurisse and Dr J. Marchand in 1918 and 1919 with pure lavender essence or with solutions containing a minimum of 2 per 1,000 of essence (sterilising dose).

Dr Bernard, of Marseille, had also noted in 1919 that the use of our hard Salvol soap with a 10% essential oil content produced remarkable results. With the lather from this soap, which, as one can imagine, has a low essential oil content, he was able to heal a post-amputation bedsore quickly which he had not previously been able to heal with any known remedy.

It seems that we now look to a formulation strikingly similar to that commonly used in cosmetics and perfumes. While these two arts have hitherto tended to use alcohol as an excipient and although this solvent is not always the ideal vehicle for medicinal uses, we note that solutions of 20 grams of essential oils per litre (good quality eau de Cologne) are ideal antiseptic liquids and, furthermore, stimulants of most of the functions which, together, constitute life itself.

This comeback of perfumery, an art too often discredited because it is "a purely sensory luxury and pleasure", and its possible use for more immediately practical purposes appears original to say the least. If nothing else, the large number of doctors, and important ones at that, who daily see the beneficial effects of the method and who use it with unabashed enthusiasm, supports the dogged work of a chemist and perfumer who has patiently endeavoured to prove the efficacy of fragrant substances.

We will cite here only a small number of observations for documentation purposes. Since 1922, the number of sick and injured people who have been healed has been so high that all have not been recorded. We will simply list some typical cases.

DR MARCHAND'S OBSERVATIONS

Excoriation on the instep of the right foot caused by the shoe. The size of a five-franc coin. Treated 31st August; healed 21st September.

Wide, infected superficial wound on the external side of the right knee: healed after two applications and one day's rest.

Infected sore on the posterior side of the instep, dating back 18 days. All the usual methods had been tried: dry and wet dressings, ointments and powders. One application of lavender. Twenty-four hours later, the sore was dry and healed. Patient was seen again 15 days later in perfect health.

Ulcerated lesion on the postero-external side of the left leg caused by an injection and dating back two months.

Three days after the first application of terpeneless lavender, the sore looked clean and was no longer festering. Patient left, healed, after one month.

Infected ulcerated lesion of the lower third of the left leg. 24th December, first application of lavender. 31st December: improvement, the purulent suppurating base was granulating and pink. By 16th January, the sore was half its original size. By 10th February, it had healed completely.

Sore on the antero-external side of the left leg. The sore was deep, gangrenous and was secreting large quantities of pus. On 31st December, the sore had not responded to any of the usual treatments. Lavender was applied and the bottom became pink, granulated and free of pus and gangrenous tissue. Dressings were hardly soiled. By 20th January, about one centimetre around the entire circumference of the sore had healed.

From 20th to 29th January, we had no lavender, cauterisation stopped and the sore remained the same and stopped improving. Treatments recommenced on the 29th, rapid progress. By 5th February, the sore was only one centimetre in diameter. Healed by the 10th.

Infected sore on the lower third of the left leg. Entered the 15th, healed the 22nd.

Wide superficial burn on the outside of the left thigh caused by mustard gas. Burned 8th September in the Aisne. Since 2nd December, small, ulcerated, excoriated, bloody spots have appeared.

Application of lavender from day one and normal dressing. Healed 31st December. Patient discharged 6th January.

Two large sores on the left leg. 24th December, first application of lavender; 31st December, sores were clean, pinkish and granulated. 16th January, sores free of gangrenous tissue and pus, but applying the essence was painful on the granulated, exposed, bloody tissue. Dressings with boiled water. 11th February, patient left healed.

DR MEURISSE'S OBSERVATIONS

Diffuse phlegmon[96] on the left buttock resulting from a clumsy injection of colloidal sulphur given by a nurse. Patient's temperature remained around 40 degrees for three days; on the day of surgery, patient's condition was not satisfactory. Operation on 7th under local anaesthesia. Ten-centimetre incision: thick yellowish pus with a penetrating odour. Washed thoroughly with a 10/1,000 solution of lavender; after washing, we found the tissue was entirely filled with pus, like a sponge.

Rapid application of pure terpeneless essence, drained with moist gauze. Temperature that evening was 38.9 degrees. The next day, the dressing was soaked with strong-smelling pus; thorough washing with 15/1,000 solution of lavender, same dressing. Temperature 37.7 degrees. On 9th, the pus did not smell as much, although large quantities were still present. We removed large yellowish clots from different parts of the abscessed area with tweezers. Temperature that evening, 37.8 degrees. Considerable sedation on 10th and following days. The oedema significantly decreased, the pus became odourless.

We continued to remove clots, but the cavity widened too quickly. Rinsed with 10/1,000 solution of lavender. 16th May, the sore was half its original size. 21st May, situation normal, healed at the end of the month.

This observation is interesting because we were able to heal a woman with a highly-infected, enormous, diffuse phlegmon in three weeks.

Fixation abscess in a patient suffering epidemic influenza with liver insufficiency. Considerable elimination of bile pigments and urobilin. Abscess on the left thigh. Opened on 9th day. Enormous gap 15 centimetres long and 9 centimetres wide. Ten-centimetre incision. A stream of odourless pus flowed out. Rinsing with 15/1,000 solution of lavender; washed the cavity with pure lavender essence; drained with wet gauze. The next day, there was a large amount of pus but it was fairly clear; elimination of gangrenous tissues. During the following days, the progress made with this treatment was unexpected because we thought it impossible for such a sore to heal without another incision in the shape of a cross. Opened on 2nd May, healed by the end of the month.

Adenophlegmon[97] on the lower left jaw. Considerable swelling around the lower left jaw, spreading to the upper hyoid area and extending beyond the left maxillary angle. Tissues hard, infiltrated, almost ligneous: a slight fluctuation could be felt; very painful when pressed. For the few days prior to the surgery, we tried intramuscular injections of colloidal silver without success.

7th June, general anaesthesia, incision; a thick, creamy pus flowed out; sterile Pasteur treatment. Deep cauterisation by thermocautery. Rinsed with lavender essence, drained with a dressing soaked in a 15/1,000 solution of essence. On the surface, wet dressing with 5/1,000 solution. Same dressing every day, but the third day, stopped rinsing with pure essence. On 14th June, we applied a zinc oxide cream with 6% essence. By 24th June, healing was complete in 16 days.

An earlier adenophlegmon, which had opened six months earlier and had been treated with oxygenated water and dilute Labarraque's solution, took 45 days to heal three centimetres; the scar remained painful and six months after the treatment, it formed another fibrous swelling surrounded by redness. Small miliary vesicles filled with pus containing staphylococci frequently appeared on the scar which was slightly keloidal.

In contrast, with the lavender essence treatment, the microscope shows rapid bacterial cleansing. The destruction of polynuclear leucocytes since their digestive role appears to have finished is shown by the fairly rapid appearance of mononuclears and even lymphocytes from the granulating tissue.

Wide contused wound on the anterior side of the thigh following an accident. Six centimetres in diameter, two centimetres deep, three days old. Base of wound was ruby red; gangrenous muscular debris, jagged edges; secreting an odorous pus. Anti-tetanus injection administered.

Cleaned the wound with warm, salted boiled water, bathed with pure terpeneless lavender essence. Packed with gauze soaked in 15/1,000 solution of essence. The pus produced a polybacterial flora with staphylococci, streptococci and thick rod-like cells with truncated ends which look like *perfringens*.

Completely healed in 34 days. The streptococci disappeared on the eighth day and the large rod-like cells had disappeared by the third day.

DR FORGUES' OBSERVATIONS

Wound on the forehead and the temporal bone area resulting from an automobile accident. Wounds on the bruised, purplish, swollen lips. The skin had detached and the muscles were severed; a haematoma was forming and was lanced; the wound reached the top of the head and extended toward the nape of the neck. Treatment: washing with four litres of water containing 5/1,000 lavender essence, drying of the wound, dry dressing. Same treatment for four days, after which time the underlying layers healed and the skin reattached. Stopped the washes, but application of 15/1,000 solution. Completely healed eight days later. Although the wound was not sutured and there was therefore a risk of infection, it nonetheless healed in twelve days.

Blow to the external condyle area of the right knee from a wood axe. The joint was intact but the blunt axe created a large wound with ragged, bruised edges which opened wide. Sutured with hair; coaptation[98] of the lips of the wound not possible. At the same time as this half-suture, thorough washing with 5/1,000 lavender solution, followed by a dry dressing. Same wash twice daily for one week. The stitches were not holding the wound together and so had to be removed. After a week, the patient was walking. The wound looked good and the underlying parts had been completely disinfected. Skin grew back rapidly and naturally. Convalescence lasted 18 days.

Hand crushed by a gunshot. The conservative method used despite the serious condition allowed the injured patient to keep a slightly deformed but functional hand. Almost continual use of 5/1,000 lavender spray and wet dressings at night.

Gangrene in the foot following a gunshot wound: Arab patient refused amputation. The accident had occurred two years previously and the patient had already lost two toes. Compresses with 15/1,000 solution produced a point of discharge along the traditional Lisfranc amputation line. The front of the foot fell off fifteen days later. Light applications to the stump healed the wound with no secondary infection.

Fistulous osteitis of the femur resulting from a gunshot wound three months earlier. Elimination of necrosed splinters and malodorous suppuration disappeared after ten days of daily instillation with 15/1,000 solution. Movement returned to the knee and the patient returned to his douar.

Colonist with ozaena.[99] Irrigations with 5/1,000 solution. After 11 days, the characteristic fetid odour disappeared.

VARICOSE ULCERS

Dr Meurisse's observations

Commercial traveller with an ulcer on the right leg dating back nine years, during which time all possible treatments had been tried with varying degrees of success, but with none healing the ulcer definitively.

No improvement for the past six months; pronounced oedema of the leg and ankles; the base of the sore was greyish, irregular elliptical shape, edges white.

Pure lavender essence applied on the base of the sore and to the edge; loose dressing with lavender-impregnated adhesive.

The sore healed 25 days later, after a number of such dressings; treated exclusively on an out-patient basis.

Prior to treatment, the microscope had revealed poly-microbial flora of an undefined type, pus globules, enlarged polynuclear leucocytes that had been or were in the process of being destroyed, and did not readily absorb the stain. Few intact polynuclear leucocytes, no mononuclears, granulated patches of cellular debris.

After the first lavender dressing: fairly large number of intact polynuclear leucocytes.

After the second dressing, proteolysis seemed complete, the bottom of the sore was already reddish; few bacteria, many cytolysed elements, few pus globules, fairly large number of mononuclears. After the third dressing, no bacteria, numerous mononuclears; after the last dressing, small amount of cellular debris, some lymphocytes and extravasated red blood cells at the point of superficial granulation.

Dr Forgues. Observation 6. Arab patient with a long-standing varicose ulcer. All else had failed. Healed in 17 days.

ATONIC WOUNDS

Dr P. Sassard's observations

Mrs S., 25 years old: torpid ulcerated lesion on the posterior side of the calf. This ulcerated lesion began with a mild scratch which was neglected and which grew considerably instead of healing. Now it was a rounded, regular, rather deep ulcerated lesion; it was not bleeding and suppurated only very slightly. Patient's general health was good and, besides a varicose state throughout the veins of the lower leg, no reason could be found for this delay in healing. For one month, we tried a wide array of treatments, but in vain; strict rest, Peru balsam ointment, zinc oxide, inotyol, mesothorium, titanium etc. A dermatologist consulted recommended that, before resigning ourselves to applying the "practitioner's bandage", we try a general treatment with local applications of pure Peru balsam and aromatic wine. This treatment proved to be as ineffective as the others. This was when, upon our advice, the patient tried lavender essence used in the following manner: careful washing of the sore with ethyl alcohol, followed by application of a small amount of lavender essence and covering with a small gauze square soaked in the same essence and held in place with tape. This dressing was changed morning and evening.

From the third day, the sore turned red and skin began to form around the edges. Healing then progressed normally and, after eight or ten days, healing was complete and continued without incident, despite patient walking and standing.

Fifty-two-year-old man burned his hand with lighted petrol. Healing, although slow, continued normally with *tulle gras* dressings changed frequently. However, for some time, despite silver nitrate, aromatic wine and other stimulants of skin growth, an anfractuous and atonic wound persisted. It was the size of a five-franc coin. Encouraged by our initial successes, we discontinued all other dressings and gave the patient three dressings a day of terpeneless lavender essence. After 48 hours, the sore started healing again and after eight days of this treatment, there remained no more than an anfractuous sore about one and a half centimetres in diameter which closed up eight days later.

Thirty-two-year-old woman: excoriation of the posterior side of the right instep. This sore was directly related to wearing a poorly-made shoe which continually hurt the patient. For a few days, the patient was forced to wear a slipper when walking and apply dressings with an insulin-based ointment. Healing did not begin and the attending physician, as an afterthought, ran a Wassermann test which was negative. We recommended the halting of all medication and all treatments except twice-daily dressings of lavender essence. Healing commenced three days after the start of this treatment and continued normally. The patient was able to walk and work again long before the sore was completely healed, although healing did progress normally.

We also obtained interesting results in cases of eczema-type dermatosis of the anterior side of the leg and varicose ulcers.

chapter six

TESTS ON THE ANTI-TOXIC ACTION OF ESSENTIAL OILS

Non-terpenic constituents of essential oils have a clear and specific activity on the production of hepatic secretions and significantly increase the production of antitoxins which enable the organism to react to the harmful action of toxic substances. However, aromatic substances themselves act as antitoxins and counteract the dangerous effects of all kinds of poisons. Ancient pharmacopoeias frequently mention the activity of aromatic substances as antigens for snake and rabid dog bites.

We have also found that only the completely volatile constituents have these properties and that, when the aromatic principles are extracted by Robiquet-Massignon processes using volatile solvents, these products of total extraction are fatal at relatively low doses (10 to 15 times less than the fatal dose of volatile oil). Finally, if the volatile constituents are removed from these extracted substances, the residues are 50 times more toxic, and sometimes even more.[100]

We were forced to conclude from this that volatile constituents greatly reduce the toxic action of products extracted by solvents and, indeed, this is what the following experiments demonstrated, the poison used being ethyl alcohol.

EXPERIMENTS

COMPARATIVE TOXICITY OF PURE ETHYL ALCOHOL AND ETHYL ALCOHOL WITH THE ADDITION OF ESSENTIAL OILS

We began our experiments by comparing the toxic effect of ordinary alcohol with that of the same alcohol with the addition of essential oils, selected from among those used in the liqueur industry: anethol from anise, fennel, lemon, bitter orange (curaçao) etc.

We used a number of guinea pigs, kept in pairs in isolated cages. In each cage, one with coloured fur was given daily an increasing dose of ethyl alcohol reduced to 30° Gay-Lussac, and a control with white fur was given the same dose of alcohol of the same titre, but with the addition of 5 parts per thousand of terpeneless essential oil.

These very healthy guinea pigs, weighing on average 400 grams, were given the following orally, to simulate real conditions as closely as possible:

for 8 consecutive days, 0.5 g of 30° G.L. alcohol
    5   1
  10   1
   5   2

After two days rest, they were sacrificed by the administration of a fatal dose of 6 grams per animal of the non-aromatised alcohol, or 7 grams of the aromatised alcohol.

From the third day, the animals treated with the non-aromatised dilute alcohol displayed the vacant facies of alcoholics: they were globular, immobile and of an absolutely characteristic appearance. The animals treated with aromatised alcohol were, on the contrary, more lively than usual: one female gave birth during the treatment without the litter showing any peculiarities and without their nursing seeming to suffer in the slightest.

On the 30th day, after two days rest, we administered the fatal dose. It should be noted that more aromatised alcohol than un-scented natural ethyl alcohol was required to kill the animals.

All the animals given aromatised alcohol urinated abundantly several times before dying. The animals treated with non-aromatised alcohol did not urinate.

When opened, we found that all the ethyl-treated animals had an extremely dilated stomach the size of a hen's egg, with peritoneal hepatic adhesions and slight ascites.[101] The liver was atrophied and cirrhotic; the biliary tract was atrophied and the Swiss tie totally relaxed. The open stomach was limp and empty; the gastric villi had completely disappeared, in particular in the large colon; the internal tunica appeared to have been completely eaten away.

These characteristics were common to all the animal treated with non-aromatised ethyl alcohol and, in fact, are in line with normal observations on all alcoholics.

In contrast, the animals treated with identical doses of alcohol of the same titre, but aromatised, did not show any special character-istics except the small white kidney found in alcoholics, with neither lesions nor adhesions. No lesion of the liver, heart or stomach. Despite the intensive 30-day alcohol regime, representing about half a litre of commercial alcohol per day for an adult human, the condition of these animals was almost normal. On the other hand, the animals treated with the same quantity of alcohol without any essence were in a very precarious state.

The animal given alcohol with fennel did have a brownish liver; this is due to the action of ketones (fenchone), an action already observed in animals treated with essential oils not dissolved in alcohol. This animal's gall bladder was slightly hypertrophied and contained a yellowish and vaguely aromatic fluid.

It is thus evident that the animals treated with the aromatised alcohol were infinitely less intoxicated than those treated with the non-aromatic alcohol. The large number of urinations, during the treatment and before death, also shows that essences have a specific action on elimination via the kidneys. During the treatment we noticed active elimination via the lungs. This elimination via the air passages obviously favours oxidation and evaporation of the alcohol, which consequently does not attach to nervous matter. Finally, the increased bile secretion, already observed with the ingestion of oil of turpentine, indicates an increase in antitoxic function.

We are thus led to the conclusion that essential oils added to a toxic product, such as alcohol, decrease its toxicity, facilitate elimination via all natural channels and counteract the toxic action due to the tonic or special action of essential oils.

These new results appear initially to contradict the observations of experts on alcoholism. In reality, this is not the case if we distinguish between alcohols which are spirits of aromatic herbs (i.e. they contain only volatile substances) and alcohols which also contain infusions and are hence alcoholic tinctures containing all the principles of extraction.

We have determined that volatile principles are not toxic, but that the action of fixed extracts is about 10 times more powerful if they still contain volatile substances, and 50 to 100 times greater if these are removed.

When Dr F. J. Collet, in his remarkable *Précis de pathologie interne* [Summary of internal pathology] tells us: "Intoxication by alcohol is inseparable from intoxication by essences; they are often chemically inseparable; this is a case of combined intoxication", it is because he does not know of this technical distinction. The alcohols he cites as dangerous are in fact not just alcohols containing essences, but alcohols containing extracts: arquebuse, absinthe, vulnerary alcoholic tincture. The distinction is, however, clearly made in the work by J. Fritsch entitled *Nouveau traité de fabrication des liqueurs* [New treatise on the manufacture of liqueurs].

Moreover, this distinction between ethyl alcoholics and liqueur alcoholics has already been made: Pierre Marie states that rural alcoholics who drink cider brandy generally die from their first crisis, due to cerebral haemorrhaging, whereas liqueur drinkers die only after a number of crises. Magnan distinguishes between the stupor of ethyl alcoholism and the euphoric stimulation caused by aromatic liqueurs. Lacassagne comments on the stupor of rural alcoholics who, although they drink less than city dwellers, absorb pure ethyl distillates. Paul, a forensic scientist from the Seine, points out that sexual performance is diminished in ethyl alcoholics but heightened in liqueur alcoholics. At the Departmental Asylum of Bron (Rhône), it was possible to compare the persistent and incurable delirium of an ethyl alcoholic and the transitory delirium of a woman intoxicated by aromatic liqueurs (Douly).

All these observations, and many more besides which there is no room to relate here, show that essential oils have a remedial and beneficial action in cases of liqueur intoxication. We would also point out that cider, wine and marc brandies generally do contain some essential oil and that the ethers which give these alcohols their bouquet are not so far removed in composition from the aromatic substances we are looking at here. However they are generally found in small quantities and their therapeutic action seems less beneficial than that of essences. The comparison would be even more favourable to essential oils if it were possible to examine subjects drinking ethyl alcohol truly devoid of aromatics, but unfortunately it is not.

Our observations fully corroborate ancient therapy and also the art of the liqueur-maker and viticulturist. Aromatic wines, spiced liqueurs and distillates of aromatic plants have always been considered to have a favourable effect, and the harmful effect of alcohol has always paled before the stimulating, carminative, diuretic, euphoric and cholagogue action of aromatic substances. That errors in application have occurred for lack of appropriate experimentation could not be more true, but these errors confirm the general rule.

PHARMACOLOGICAL CONSEQUENCES

From a therapeutic standpoint, the consequences of these observations are considerable.

The French Codex distinguishes between spirits of aromatic herbs, which contain only the volatile elements, and alcoholic tinctures which contain both the essence and the extract. Distilled vulnerary spirit is not confused with vulnerary alcoholic tincture, which is used particularly for aromatic wine for external use. Spirits and alcoholic tinctures of star aniseed must not be used indiscriminately any more than should spirits and alcoholic tinctures of lemon, bitter orange etc.

On the other hand, certain aromatic plant extracts prepared by boiling with water contain only the soluble substances in the liquid. The volatile elements are eliminated during distillation (boiling or concentration). These extracts are more toxic and less effective than if the eliminated volatile elements were returned to them. The dosage could conceivably be higher without reaching a toxic level on the one hand, and, on the other, the essential oil would contribute its therapeutic effect to that of the extract. Finally, the presence of the antiseptic essence in the extract would doubtless mean that it would keep longer. In discussing plant extracts in his *Cours de Chimie* [Lessons in chemistry], Paris 1675, Nicolas Lémery expressly states: "this preparation is good for mixtures which do not have an odour. It is not the same for those that do, for evaporation removes the best part, namely the volatile. Thus I do not advise anyone to make extracts from aromatics."

Quincy, an English doctor in the early nineteenth century, expressed the same reservations and reaffirmed Lémery's indications, stressing them in his *Pharmacopoeia Officinalis et extemporanea*. "This is how extraction is normally done" he says, "but its use in medicine does not seem to be as great as is generally imagined for all the most subtle particles escape and dissipate; the menstruum is either removed by distillation or evaporates into the air" (quoted by Adrian. *Etude historique sur les extraits pharmaceutiques* [Historical study of pharmaceutical extracts], Paris 1889).

On the subject of his plant salts, De La Garaye (1745) states: "Decoction and infusion are useless for . . . aromatic plants, as they thereby lose their ethereal oil and their volatile salt" (De La Garaye, *Chimie Hydraulique pour extraire les sels essentiels des végétaux* [Hydraulic chemistry for extracting essential salts from plants], Paris 1745).

These categorical reserves, which clearly indicate that experts considered essential oils to be the most valuable and effective substances in aromatic plants, could well be repeated today since vacuum evaporation methods do not eliminate the risk of the almost total loss of volatile elements.

PRACTICAL CONSEQUENCES

TABLE LIQUEURS

Early liqueurs were always aromatic solutions and were primarily used for the health and for therapeutic purposes. The first fermented drinks were wines into which aromatic or medicinal plants were infused: aloe, aniseed, hyssop, myrrh, rosemary, sage. These "herbal wines", which Grégoire de Tours calls "Vina Odoramentis Immixta" were generally considered to be remedies but subsequently passed over into general consumption. Thirteenth century poets speak of them rapturously, as being delicious and indispensable at festivities of any kind.

True liqueurs were invented by monks in the thirteenth and fourteenth centuries. One of the first, attributed to collaboration between Arnault de Villeneuve and Raymond Lulle, was made of brandy, sugar and aromatics, such as lemon, roses, orangeflower etc.

The liqueurs of fifteenth-century Florence, Venice and Turin have not been ousted by modern creations and the origins of the cultivation of aromatics in northern Italy lie in this industry. The "populo" famous in the times of the Medicis was fragranced with amber, musk, aniseed and cinnamon. Louis XIV certainly had a taste for liqueurs which, it is said, gave him his vigour in old age.

The liqueurs of Montpellier and Lorraine enjoyed great popularity. Maraschino, over which the Senate of Venice had a monopoly, the cordial of Collandon, a doctor in Geneva, and Curaçao from the Dutch colonies were all strongly fragranced alcohols, the stimulant properties of which were never at issue and doctors always recommended them.

The popular spirits of today are rakis, mastics, aniseed spirits and gins, with more people drinking them by far than non-aromatic alcohols.

Aniseed and its liqueurs, about which so much has been written, have been consumed all around the Mediterranean for centuries without incident: Hippocrates, Theophrastus, Dioscorides and Columella recommended the use of aniseed as a stomachic stimulant. The fact that, in his *Capitularies*, Charlemagne recommended the cultivation of aniseed, and famous Arab doctors prepared efficacious remedies from it to fight sciatica and intestinal diseases, demonstrates that aniseed is not a dangerous substance – indeed quite the contrary. Pliny the Elder asserted that aniseed causes mild drowsiness, gives a freshness to the face and reduces wrinkles. H. Blin recently said that aniseed stimulates the stomach, enlivens the circulation and transforms and protects mucous membranes from a catarrhal state. Regular use of aniseed alleviates malaria. Forgues says that it clearly disinfects the stomach and intestines, even in cases of colibacillosis. Reutter, although no devotee of essences, states that, like orangeflower water, aniseed slows the heartbeat slightly while increasing the number of leucocytes in the blood and stimulating the secretion of saliva and bile. Essence of aniseed kills *Eberthella typhosa*, staphylococcus and diphtheria bacilli within 24 hours, and meningococcus within one hour (Morel and Rochaix). Senator Grosjean reported numerous cases of cholera healed by a vicar apostolic in Cochin China in 1912 using aniseed-flavoured liqueurs. Varenne, J. Roussel and Godefroy demonstrated that essence of aniseed is never toxic, even in very high doses, and that because of its chemical composition, it is analgesic and antiseptic. Dr Dalou stated that, at a dose of 3 grams per kilograms animal body weight, it has never caused any toxic incident.

These time-honoured practices generally have a solid experimental foundation resulting from thousands of observations.

On the basis of our experiments, we will henceforth make a clear distinction between spirits of aromatic herbs, such as anisette, white curaçao, peppermint and so on, which are entirely volatile, and alcoholic tinctures based on infusions or extracts of plants, peels etc. In addition to distilled spirits of herbs, absinthe, now banned, contained plants infusions, in particular those of wormwood, hyssop or rue, tansy etc. Infusions of these plants are toxic, whereas their volatile essences are not.[102]

We would say that when a liqueur is mentioned by name by an expert as being dangerous, it is in most cases a liqueur containing infusions and not a pure distillate.[103]

THE CYTOPHYLACTIC[104] POWER OF ESSENCES

While not in any way underestimating the importance of the antiseptic power of essences, it appears from the observations we have published that this is not the only property behind the rapid healing of wounds.

At the start of treatment, rapid bacteriolysis[105] together with the destruction of excess extravasated polynuclears is, as Dr Meurisse reports, certainly witnessed. However, in cases where the wounds are not bacterial and suppuration is insignificant or non-existent, what is it that "triggers" the healing of a wound which had hitherto remained atonic and not responded to any of the usual medication?

Lymph afflux, rapid proteolysis by the release of leucocytic ferments, explains Dr Meurisse . . . this triggering of phenomena by an aromatic substance (for many essences have the same action as lavender) closely resembles the power of certain vitamins and animal hormones.

It must therefore be conceded that, while the antiseptic power of essences is of enormous interest, especially since it is not attended by any of the disadvantages found to such a large degree with all the other antiseptics used hitherto, greater attention needs to be devoted to the power they have of vitalising tissue.

As the use of pure essential oil of lavender seems to us difficult and awkward in certain cases, we have studied new dilutions in soapy excipients and found that it is totally futile to use the pure essences. The same dynamic effects on cells are obtained at a high dilution. Sapolinol, for example, is a special soapy liquid containing just 4% of selected essential oils, one of which is lavender. Dr P. Sassard, who conducted the initial tests on it, declares that Sapolinol demonstrates its full power on infected and atonic wounds.

a) Wounds sustained in accidents: cuts, scratches, scalps.

b) Abscesses, phlegmons, whitlows, cold abscesses become inflamed etc.; usually in addition to surgical treatment.

c) Burns, regardless of depth and extent. As the product is neither toxic nor caustic, it can be applied liberally, even to large areas of bleeding. It has an analgesic, disinfectant and above all a highly cicatrisant effect. Normalisation of healing is characteristic: keloids and adhesive scars are avoided, factors of particular relevance for facial burns.

d) Wounds to the bones or joints: there is no reason why an aromatic solution cannot be introduced into the seat of a fracture or a joint cavity: Carrel irrigation is absolutely indicated.

e) Morbid infected wounds. They are cleaned and deodorised immediately and the inflammatory infectious element is reduced to a minimum. The anus can be easily cleaned and deodorised by enema with a 10% solution.

f) Atonic wounds to limbs, delayed healing after an operation. When a wound halts during the normal healing process and, even without any additional infectious factor, becomes atonic, aromatic dressings are marvellously effective. With a 50% solution, the wound vascularises once more, the flesh returns to a healthy red colour and epidermisation is evident again.

This type of treatment is to be recommended in all cases of atonic wounds to the head or limbs, or to promote the healing of operative wounds which are slow to heal (hernia with consecutive haematoma, suppurative and largely drained appendicitis, abscesses, incised phlegmons with only a slight tendency to heal etc.).

g) Originally atonic wounds: bedsores, leg ulcers, fistulas, cavities of cold abscesses etc.

The vitality of tissues constituting the seat of the wound change rapidly and healing is rapid, even if the atonia lasts for years. Here are some more recent observations (Dr P. Sassard, *Bulletin médical* [Medical Bulletin], Feb. 1932):

> Wounds to the scalp: healed in 10 days;
> Phylctenoid[106] whitlow on the right thumb: healed in 3 days;
> Infected herpes vesicle: healed in 5 days;
> Suppurating haematoma: healed in 10 days;
> Lime burn: healed in 20 days;
> Firearm wound: healed in 15 days;
> Sacral bedsore due to a thigh fracture in a 68-year-old woman: healed in 11 days;
> Crushing of the thigh, open leg fracture;
> Varices becoming ulcerated; delayed healing of an amputation stump of the thigh: healed in 21 days after failing with all other medication; various ulcer.

In all cases, the following is noted:
rapid disappearance of pus;
decrease in the number of bacteria;
powerful stimulation of healing;
recovery in a very short time.

It is as though the physiological matter receives an added dynamism causing the pathological phenomena to abate immediately. This is the normal mechanism of the action of vitamins and hormones.

We thus have reason to regard essential oil treatments as a new "plant hormone" therapy which is certainly original and hitherto unsuspected.

THE SCENTED DRESSING

In 1912, Dr A. Cartaz reported on the benefits of fragranced bandages in an article that appeared in *La Nature* [Nature]. He stated that Dr Championnière – who can rightly be considered the father of antisepsis in France – turned some time ago to balms and essences in his search for safe antiseptic preparations. Guided by Chamberland's wonderful work, he used these fragranced principles with success.

M. Even, a pharmacist and former student of Championnière, acting on his recommendations, impregnated gauze with essential oils such as geranium, rosemary, lavender and bergamot. These volatile oils were selected not because of their pleasant odour, but because, in his opinion, they had the greatest antiseptic value while being the least irritating.

The gauze thus prepared was absolutely sterile. Placed on the skin, even in large quantities, its local or medicinal action was no more pronounced than plain gauze, but it did have an advantage: it could be impregnated with serum, blood and other fermentable matter without any fermentation or infection occurring for a period of several days. Even's gauze thus had true antiseptic value. Dr Championnière used these dressings in a wide range of circumstances, and, in every case, they afforded admirable protection.

In his conclusion, Dr Cartaz stated that the use of this fragranced gauze would be worthwhile, but its use does not appear to have increased since 1912.

This could be due to a number of reasons. Firstly, the essences impregnating ordinary gauze oxidise quite rapidly and thus some of their action is lost. Secondly, gauzes fragranced in this way do not wet as readily so-called "hydrophilic" gauzes and, if they are intended not to be moistened, it is preferable to impregnate them with a fatty or waxy substance to preserve the properties of the essential oils by preventing their oxidation. Gauzes and *tulle gras* do not adhere to wounds and, when dressings are changed, do not cause the painful tearing off of tissue being formed, which prolongs cicatrisation and irritates the underlying tissue.

This explains why *tulle gras* and waxy products such as ambrine have replaced aromatic gauzes.

In 1918, Dr Forgues reported on a type of fatty dressing which could be used like ambrine, but without the need to melt it. His formula was as follows:

Terpeneless essence of lavender .... 3 grams
Anhydrous lanolin 12   "
White petrolatum, q.s. for 45   "

He used this ointment in numerous cases, adding zinc oxide, bismuth nitrate, mercury ointment, methyl salicylate etc., depending upon the circumstances.

Fatty substances, however, have the disadvantage of completely isolating a wound from the ambient air, allowing only anaerobic fermentation to take place, yet it is becoming ever more certain that a wound which is healing needs oxygen. Experience proves that the air filtering through a fragranced membrane becomes not only perfectly aseptic, but even antiseptic. This is why, in 1918, I prepared a wide-mesh tulle impregnated with a special mixture of plastic and aromatised waxes. The air, slowly passing through this tulle, was impregnated with the vapours of essences and became antiseptic. A tulle prepared in this way does not adhere to wounds any more than does a *tulle gras*, but it is cleaner and can be handled without soiling the hands, gloves, instruments or even the wound itself, which it nonetheless keeps in an acceptable state of positive asepsis. Oxidation of the aromatic substances is prevented by the plastic composition, which acts as an anti-oxidant. The strips or pieces of tulle can be kept in a sealed jar for several years without deterioration.

Recent experiments by Dr F . . ., the head of a laboratory in a Parisian hospital, have demonstrated that the mere presence of a filter paper saturated with 4 drops of selected essences, in a container holding 10 litres of air, is sufficient to sterilise the air. While laboratory air normally spawns 100 colonies per 10 litres (or 10,000 colonies per cubic metre) before fragrancing, the same air, when fragranced, contains but 6,000 germs after 20 minutes contact with the 4 drops of essences, 2,000 germs after one hour, 1,000 germs after 3 hours, and 0 after 9 hours contact.

Certain essences act more slowly if their diffusion in the air is less prompt or less abundant, while others act more quickly in the opposite case or if the air is forced through the fragranced filter. If the quantity and quality of the essence are appropriate, antisepsis is practically guaranteed. We can assume that the gases emanating from volatile oils act on the wound itself and penetrate its smallest cracks and crevices, so that in a matter of hours a wound covered with an aromatic waxed tulle becomes aseptic and remains in this state as long as the air reaching it does so only through the aromatic mesh. Not only are outside microbes entering destroyed, but fermentation is delayed and germs from the internal infection are destroyed as they reach the area of fragranced air.

This way of using essential oils could possibly allow the most powerful constituents, phenols, to be used, provided they do not come into direct contact with the tissues, or the most volatile ones, such as terpenes, to be used without causing any irritation.

The sterility of ordinary gauze used in dressings is completely negative. That is, the bandages cease to be sterile as soon as they come in contact with the outside air, the dust in which, as Dr Fraenkel's experiments show, contains a large number of colonies per cubic metre. In contrast, a piece of hydrophilic gauze kept in a box with a bottom made of a square of essence-based waxed tulle remains "positively" aseptic during use as long as it remains impregnated with aromatic vapours.

BALNEOLOGY

The highly remarkable properties of essential oils indicate their use in balneology. Absorption of the fragrant plant "hormones" through the entire surface of the skin is an excellent means to success.

Oil of turpentine or pine extracts have often been used in baths. Turpentine can be beneficial to certain skin diseases as it increases the speed of desquamation of the scales of skin already becoming detached.

Essences of fir, pumilio pine and spruce, which contain more active elements such as borneol, bornyl acetate, cedrol etc., undoubtedly act in a different way. Cutaneous absorption is greater than generally thought, especially if the essence is perfectly diffused in water[107] and if the water contains salts to make it suitably hypotonic. Resinous baths are used to counter rheumatism, especially where followed by massage with a cream, ointment or liquid containing more active substances.

Coriander, cajeput, hyssop, oregano and sassafras are recommended as sudorifics. For balneology, the formulae of Professor Fabre, of Lyon, can be used:

Formula I. Oil of turpentine .... 25 cc
Tincture of quillaia .... 5 "
Distilled water .... 600 "

Mix and agitate. However, this emulsion separates in hot water. It is preferable to use:

Formula III. 50% sodium sulphoricinate .... 125 cc
              Oil of turpentine 15
and then to add:
              Distilled water, q.s. for .... 300 "
              Sodium borate powder .... 20 "
The solution must always contain an excess of sodium borate.

Under no circumstances do we recommend preparations containing formol, the tanning effect of which is bad for the epidermis and dangerous for the mucous membranes.

Like us, Dr Boucher of Avignon prefers the sulphoricinate formula we have been recommending since 1909 for the emulsification of all essential oils.

The dose of 300 grams can hardly be exceeded in a bath, but a 15-gram dose of turpentine appears inadequate in most cases. As matters now stand, it is very easy to introduce 100 or even 200 grams of essences into a 300-gram dose for a bath.[L] However, this dose is not worthwhile if active products such as borneol, bornyl ethers, terpineol, fenchone and other substances found in essences of conifer needles are used.

The essences of angelica, lovage or wild mountain celery, parsley, sassafras, sandalwood and many others are diuretic. Floral essences, which are more pleasant for balneology, are also beneficial, but too few tests have yet been conducted to determine their specific properties. Whilst we are perfectly aware, in our work, that all work to date should form the subject of extensive testing which will profoundly change current ideas, Dr Forgues does, nevertheless, state that carnation is carminative; rose, eupeptic; fern, diuretic and emetic; lilac, purgative and cholagogue; violet, soporific; and jasmine, stimulant. We believe that the sensitivity of individuals to fragrances differs and can even depend on an individual's own odiferous emanations. This is why the information above is valid only as preliminary experience requiring further study.

Twenty-five years of sporadic experimentation in no way constitutes a monument of certainty. In this field more than in any other, time alone will enable reliable knowledge to be established.

ESSENTIAL OILS IN DENTAL SURGERY

The information given on the use of essences and their constituents in surgery apply equally to dental surgery. All essential oils and aromatic substances in general can be considered as excellent antiseptics and powerful aids to healing; they are analgesic, antipyogenic and generally not irritant at effective doses.[108]

For mouthwashes in particular, dentists have used all the known antiseptics – benzoic acid, boric acid, salicylic acid, β-naphthol, mercuric bichloride and potassium permanganate – without realising that these highly soluble substances should be immediately rejected as the patient cannot keep them in his mouth long enough for them to take effect.

Aromatic products, on the other hand, "perfume" the mouth for hours and, as has been proven beyond doubt, they produce a more lasting effect, thus increasing the chances of truly effective elimination of germs.

Menthol and essence of mint, combined with the essences of anise (or anethol), clove (or eugenol), cinnamon etc. are used for these mouthwashes either in alcohol solutions diluted with water (for use as dental elixirs), in glycerine-based pastes (toothpastes), in powders, or in solid or preferably liquid soaps.

If astringents, such as rhatany or pyrethrum root extracts, tincture of benzoin etc., are added to these mixtures, they produce solutions which fulfil theoretical requirements and, curiously enough, these solutions are precisely those created by perfumers by an empiricism remarkable both for its foresight and its accuracy, well before the antiseptic power of essences was officially acknowledged. As a result, the most frequently used toothpastes have an undeniable worth and leave little room for improvement.

However, dental surgery properly speaking has a number of requirements which even the best toothpastes cannot fulfil as, once the nerve, or pulp, is removed, a tooth only appears to be alive. In reality it is dead and must be treated as such. It must be embalmed, to use our previous terminology, or, more exactly, it must be treated mechanically and therapeutically so that the substance of which the tooth is made cannot further deteriorate.

Generally, the excitation of the nerve of a tooth is due to some degree of deterioration: part of the tissue, enamel, dentine and cement is destroyed as a result of the effect of various anaerobic microorganisms, and sometimes an abscess even forms at the apex. First and foremost, the seats of infection must be eliminated by the application of powerful antiseptics.

These antiseptics are sometimes phenols – cresols, carbolic acid, eugenol, guaiacol etc. – or aldehydes – formalin and its derivatives being the most commonly used of these.

Phenols are necrosing agents, which means that they soften the tissue being destroyed and it can thus be removed surgically. However, they should not really be allowed to act on healthy tissue and nor should they be applied to mucous membranes which they would also destroy.

Formol and trioxymethylene, in contrast, are tanning and sclerosing agents. Tissue impregnated with formol or its vapours become hard and horny.

Eugenol (a constituent extracted from either essence of clove or cinnamon leaf) is without doubt the least caustic phenol and that best tolerated by the mucous membranes. Its odour and taste are not unbearable and considerably less unpleasant than those of the phenols from coal distillates (phenol and cresol). This is why eugenol is increasingly preferred.

Thymol is hardly ever used and carvacrol is seldom used except in mixtures as patients tend to dislike the taste of thyme.

Of the aromatic aldehydes, only cinnamic aldehyde can be used. It has almost all the antiseptic qualities of eugenol, but it is neither a necrosing nor caustic substance and its warm flavour combines well with the flavours of other essences or constituents which can be used, such as geraniol and citronellol, or geranium essence in which they are found.

Antiseptic products sold to dentists are often empirical mixtures containing various phenols, cresol, guaiacol and eugenol, and even formol, all of them aromatised and supplemented by rose essences which are rich in geraniol and citronellol, substances which smell pleasant and, as demonstrated by Paul Courmont, have antiseptic properties.

Nevertheless, phenols and formol should not be used together. Their incompatibility translates into rapid resinification and disappearance of the aldehyde for various reasons.

Nonetheless, the root canal and the cavity beyond the apex are quite often disinfected with mixtures of this sort. A dressing impregnated with the antiseptic liquid is introduced into the canal which has been widened with a drill. The antiseptic acts with varying degrees of speed either by contact or by the vapours it releases.

If the underlying cavity is infected and irritated, the formol vapours dry out the tissue forming insoluble "residues" which are difficult to reabsorb subsequently and which can cause problems in the future. Phenol vapours, which do not cause hardening, are less troublesome, and those of equally effective essences, with a clearly demonstrated cytophylactic power, are always preferable. Tests conducted with terpeneless lavender essence have shown that in most cases perfect antisepsis was achieved and the healing of damaged tissue was fast and complete with no hardening or irritation. On the other hand, lavender does not help to eliminate the carious parts of the tooth.

The taste of lavender essence does not seem to be favourably received by patients so it is a good idea to mix it with more pleasantly flavoured essences. New antiseptic preparations can therefore be much more varied than has hitherto been thought possible, without any loss in their efficacy.

Where a dressing has to be applied rapidly and cannot be changed frequently, the cavity created by the drill can be filled if not permanently, then at least temporarily. Under no circumstances must saliva be allowed to penetrate the dressing or pathogenic germs will be reintroduced into the defenceless tissue. The property phenols have of forming cements with metal oxide is used for temporary fillings of this kind.

Zinc oxide moistened with eugenol forms a mastic which can be introduced into the root canal or into cleaned cavities and which hardens them. The filling thus made with a hard, permanent product leaves a powerful antiseptic in place which continues to work on the areas susceptible to infection.

Zinc eugenate usually contains one part of uncombined eugenol, the smell of which is recognisable after a long period of time. Cement sets at a speed which varies depending on whether a light or heavy zinc oxide is used and whether it was made with water. There are various hardening accelerators which, with a particular oxide, can make cement set more quickly.

Zinc eugenate can also be used for making highly accurate impressions and several dental specialities are based on this property.

Essences and their constituents must gradually replace carbolic acid and cresylic acids both in dental surgery and in other types of surgery even though the use of cresols is less problematic on bony tissue than on any other live tissue.

Mouthwashes with essences and concentrated liquids sold commercially need to take greater account of the dosage indicated by laboratory tests. The power of aromatic solutions of elixirs is often close to the level at which the sterilising strength can no longer be observed.

We should also take account of the effect of soaps on secretions in the mouth. Much more thorough cleansing and greatly improved asepsis are achieved with soap-based washes than with washes made from alcohol solutions.

THE TOXICITY OF ESSENTIAL OILS

M ost authors on this subject speak of the toxicity of essential oils as if it were common knowledge. Even we ourselves, on the basis of what we had been taught (Eulenberg), regarded nitrobenzene as a dangerous product, but when we were able to experiment with it, we found that this product, with a formula similar to that of the dangerous substance cyanogen, is almost completely harmless. All we achieved by intramuscular injection was remarkable analgesia, followed, when we increased the dosage, by a state of stupor comparable to a uraemic coma. Like all nitro-substances, nitrobenzene (essence of mirbane) thus induces a particular intoxication, but at substantial doses of as much as 2 grams per kilogram animal body weight.

We had occasion to perform this test on a dog whose hindquarters had been crushed by an automobile. Immediately after the injection, the pain stopped completely and the dog dragged itself, by its front paws, over to lick its master and showed no signs of pain, although it did subsequently have to be destroyed.

We are therefore justified in believing that much of the information regarding the toxicity of essential oils is based "on tradition" and has not been tested recently.[110]

In this work, we have given a number of examples of conclusive experiments. In particular, the injection of alcoholic liquids containing essences has demonstrated that, far from adding one toxic power to another toxic power, essential oils in fact reduce the harmful action of the alcohol.

In most cases of poisoning, the essences acted mechanically by asphyxia, for example where doses were such that elimination via the lungs was not rapid enough and localisation in the lungs forced out the physiological liquids, by halting the exchange of gases; or, where elimination was not rapid enough, the volatile liquids, solvents of fats, became fixed in the pathways or the nerve centres. All this occurred at doses at which, in these conditions, most normal products become toxic.

This was not the case, as we have said, with the non-volatile products found with essential oils when plants or flowers are extracted with volatile solvents. However, these are no longer volatile products, but fixed impurities which need to be removed in order to remain within the strict definition of the substances concerned here.

Terpenes can have a certain irritating power and, if ingested, can dissolve the mucous membrane which prevents the auto-digestion of the membranes of the digestive tract. Phenols have a necrosing power, but to a lesser degree than phenols extracted from coal distillates, which are clearly caustic.

Nevertheless, we cannot ignore the teachings of Simon and Mitscherlich which must be based on methodical experiments. According to these authors, a certain number of essences such as anise, wormwood, lemon and orangeflower, cause congestion and inflammation of the intestines.[111] It is true that Varenne, Godefroy and Roussel affirm (and we have tested it) that anethol and anise pose no risk. Lemon, which contains 95% terpenes by weight, can dissolve mucin quite readily; orangeflower essence is sedative and hypnotic according to Grégoire, but these contradictory statements cannot constitute a basis for any definite stance.

Professor H. Bottu, professor of toxicology at the Medical School of Reims, tells us (*Parfumerie Moderne*, January 1910) that, of all the essential oils, raw natural essence of bitter almonds is the most dangerous because it contains hydrocyanic acid. We do indeed believe that hydrocyanic acid is particularly toxic wherever it is found, but that it constitutes only an impurity which is easily eliminated from the commercial essence.[112]

The natural essence without the hydrocyanic acid, adds Bottu, and likewise the synthetic essence, are not toxic.[113]

Juniper essence is said to be the second most toxic oil after the above.[114] Juniper essence normally contains 75% terpenes by weight. It would take 30 grams to induce any incident. There is no question that absorption of 21 grams of pinene or oil of turpentine corresponding to this "weight of juniper essence" would pose some risk. This is what seems to emerge from the rest of the text: "it increases urinary secretions and makes the urine smell of violets *like oil of turpentine* . . . It causes haematemesis and diarrhoea; the kidneys are bloated with blood". This is precisely the effect of a high dose of turpentine.[115]

Mr Bottu then tells us that ketonic essences are dangerous (fennel, caraway, savin), abortive and cause generalised clogging of the blood vessels in the stomach and the intestines without causing inflammation or congestion in the jejunum. Our own observations add "clear adverse effect on the liver".[116]

Certain treatises classify geranium, star anise, eucalyptus and cajeput essences as toxic . . . Thirty grams of clove essence is said to cause "loss of consciousness". Does anise oil, which attracts fish, really act as a neuro-narcotic on these animals?[117]

Reutter states in all seriousness that all essences cause nausea and migraines and he records these effects, which are purely mental and personal, as a proof of toxicity. Nothing of the sort has ever been observed in factories where essential oils are handled by the ton or in perfumeries where "industrial" accidents are never due to the perfumes.

Stories by neurologists that society women surrounded by perfumes are subject to nervous disorders are nothing more than fabrications.

Crystallised vanillin, like benzoic acid, can cause certain types of eczema, but this skin irritation is caused by extremely fine acicular crystals which penetrate the epidermis like the stinging hairs of nettles and cause a particular kind of irritation. Even then, the phenomenon is purely physical and quickly stops when the cause, the handling of the crystallised substance, is removed.

Thujone (ketone) is toxic (F. Jurss, 1903) and myristicin too, apparently. Safrole is thought to cause degeneration of the fatty tissue of the liver and kidneys.[118]

In reality, the very relative toxicity of essential oils tends principally to prove their physiological action. If we deduce from our experiments, conducted with great care over a long period of time, that this toxicity is reduced almost to zero when constituents with known harmful effects (terpenes and, in certain cases, ketones) or dangerous impurities (fixed extracts, hydrocyanic acid) are removed, we can see that essential oils are relatively very safe active substances which are suitable for many therapeutic applications.

CONCLUSIONS

I s it not too early to draw conclusions from this objective account? Our early works resulted in thousands of tests, generated new verification procedures and gave rise to numerous effective remedies. The results obtained attest to the therapeutic value of aromatic substances. Remedies using essences already help many patients and save many lives.

The future will determine the position which aromatic substances are to hold in new pharmacopoeias.

In the meantime, it is possible to formulate some hypotheses about the way they act.

The chemical action is beyond us, as is the chemical action of most of the remedies already in use, but chemistry is gradually moving toward physics, and physics provides us with some interesting hypotheses.

Essential oils (and especially their oxygenised constituents) alter the surface tension of liquids, are soluble in lipids, have a high absorptive power and are highly permeable (K. W. Rosenmund, *Angewandte Chemie* [Applied Chemistry], 45.7.1935). They are used in industry as wetting agents and their presence in water profoundly transforms its properties. When suspended in blood, particles of essences sometimes gather on the walls of vessels or on the surface of blood corpuscles, radically altering their tension and permeability. Snake venom and some viruses act via a similar mechanism but in the opposite direction. Old pharmacopoeias recommended aromatic substances as antidotes for snake venom and for the rabies virus, perhaps because they act in exactly the opposite direction, albeit in the same way.

Essences are likely to prevent certain flocculations[119] and reduce the effect of shock. When used to dissolve or dilute substances to be injected, they prevent some incidents and reinforce the effect of certain substances.

However, in addition to this generic action, essential oils all act in specific ways.

Every aromatic constituent has a particular electromagnetic composition (P. Debeye, *Polare Molekeln* [Polar Molecules], Leipzig, 1929, and Arno Müller, *Parfumerie Moderne* 145, 1936). Perfume molecules are highly polarised and this polarisation, accentuated in dilution, explains the action of dilute solutions. The particular excitation of each dipolar molecule is translated, in the olfactory nerve, by differing sensations of smell and, in tissue and body fluids, by local changes in magnetic fields due to polarity neutralisation or reversals.

This property, particular to aromatic substances and not shared by other substances, explains their superiority. The changing of relationships between cells, blood corpuscles, lipids and salts themselves and all colloids with each other and with physiological fluids; the transformation of polarities and magnetic fields; what more can be needed to attest to the activity of these substances which are, in addition, safe?

What other products, chemical or natural, can offer such tremendous potential?

An initial series of experiments is now completed and the systematic study is beginning. We are happy to have been the first to envisage and to use the therapeutic properties of aromatic substances and we hope they have an illustrious future.[120]

With our laboratories and our specialised production, we remain at the disposal of all researchers.

BIBLIOGRAPHY

1680   Matthiole. Commentaires de Dioscorides. A du Pinet. Lyon.

1694   Pomet. Histoire Générale des Drogues. Paris.

1773   J. F. Demachy. L'art du Distillateur des eaux fortes. Paris.

1796   Carmichael. An account of the experiment. Cité par Guyton de Morveau, Nouveau Traité des moyens de désinfecter l'air. Paris, An IX.

1798   Lémery. Dictionnaire Universel des Drogues simples. V. Houry. Paris.

An VII   Racaché Joseph B. Réflexions sur les odeurs. Thèse de Montpellier.

An XII   Buchoz. Monographie de la rose et de la violette. Paris.

1811   Galesio. Traité des Citrus. Paris.

1812   Virey. Des Odeurs que répandent les animaux. Bull. de Pharmacie.

1813   Risso. Essai sur l'Histoire naturelle des Orangers. Paris.

1818   Risso et Poiteau. Histoire naturelle et culture des orangers, 2° Ed. du Breuil. 1872.

1821   H. Cloquet. Osphrésiologie ou Traité des Odeurs. Paris.

1873   Chatin Johannès. Recherches sur les glandes odorantes des mammifères. Ann. des sc. Nat. Paris.

1874   Goeze. Bertrag zur Kentniss des Orengervachse. Hamburg.

1874   Robinet. Thèse. Ecole de Pharmacie de Paris.

1875   Husemann. Arch. für exptl. Path. u. Pharm. 4.280.

1887   Chamberland. Ann. de l'Inst. Pasteur. 153.

1888   Voiry. Thèse. Paris.

1888   Cadéac et Albin Meunier. Recherches expérimentales sur l'action antiseptique des essences. Ann. Inst. Pasteur Ill. 188.

1889   Blondel. Les produits odorants du sorier. Paris.

1890   Nannotti. Recherches expérimentales et cliniques sur l'action de l'essence de girofle dans les affections tuberculeuses. Semaine médicale.

1890   Semmler. Sur la myristicine. D. Chem. H. XXII. 1803.

1890   John Maisch. A manual of organic materia medica 4° ed.

1891   Cadéac et A. Meunier. Note sur les propriétés épileptisantes de l'essence d'hysope. Soc. de Biol.

1893   Bertrand. Le Gomenol. Bull. Gén. de Thér. Ann. de l' I. Pasteur.

1893   Huchard. Revue générale de clinique et thérapeutique.

1893   Hallopeau. Sur le traitement de la pelade par l'essence de Wintergreen. Soc. de Dermatologie.

1893   De la Jarrige. Injections massives intra-pulmonaires d'huile créosotée et mentholée. Congrès pour l'étude de la Tuberculose.

1893   Bouchard et Oliviero. Bull. Soc. Chim. de Paris.

1894   Charrin. Action des essences sur le microbe du Choléra. Soc. Biol.

1895   Zwaardemaker. Physiologie des Geruchs. Leipzig.

1895   Dujardin-Beaumetz et Maire. Bull. Gén. de Thérapeutique.

1896   Letanneur. Thérapeutique médicale.

1896   Alp. de Candolle. Origine des plantes cultivées. Paris 4° éd.

1898   Dubousquet Laborderie. Communication sur les applications thérapeutiques du Goménol. Soc. de Thérapeutique.

1898   Tardif Etienne. Etude critique des Odeurs, Thèse de Bordeaux.

1898   Raphaël Dubois. Le sens olfactif de l'escargot. C. R. Soc. de Biol. 198.

1899   1900. L. Trabut. Sur l'huile de cèdre de l'Atlas. Bull. Soc. Pharm. t. 1.262.

1901   H. Huertas. Le Cèdre en thérapeutique. Thèse Méd. Montpellier.

1901   P. Brunet-Manquat. Produits retirés du cèdre et leur emploi en médecine. Bull. Méd. de l'Algérie 12ᵉ an. 151.

1901   Beauregard. Matière médicale zoologique. Naud. Paris.

1902   Guegen. Pouvoir antiseptique du Goménol.

1902   Fromm et Hildebrand. Destinée des terpènes et complexes cycliques dans l'organisme. Bull. Soc. Chim. France 28. 190 et 1903 30–658.

1902   Hildebrandt. Arch. f. Exptl. Path. 48.451.

1903   Arnozan. Précis de thérapeutique; t. 1.

1903   Ant. Combes. Influence des parfums sur les néyropathes, thèse de Bordeaux.

1904   G. Jougla. Contribution à l'étude chimique, toxicologique et thérapeutique des essences. Thèse Paris.

1904   Fromm et Clémens. Réaction du Sabinol dans l'organisme. Bull. Soc. Ch. de France 32. 1066 et 1149.

1904   E. Varenne. Etudes sur l'anéthol et l'estragol. Thèse de pharm. Paris.

1905   Odeurs et troubles cardiaques. Paris.

1906   Lesieur. Ch. Nouvelles recherches expérimentales sur la toxicité des essences usuelles. Ann. de Méd. expér. et analyt. T. XVIII, 801.

1906   Hérail. Traité de pharmacologie et matière médicale.

1906   Kettenkoffen. P. L'Ylang Ylang. Thèse de Bonn.

1907   Hildebrandt. Neuere Arzneimittel. 145.

1907   Rigaux. Le Goménol. Thérapeutique chirurgicale. Thèse Lyon.

1907   Péju. A propos de l'action bactéricide de l'essence de téré benthine. Soc. de Biol.

1908   Rolland. Flore Populaire. Paris.

1908   Guégen. Pouvoir antiseptique et bactéricide du Goménol, Soc. de Biol.

1908 et 1911   Ellis Havelock. Etude de psychologie sexuelle.

1908   Desgrez. Innocuité du Goménol.

1908   Cabanès. Bull. Gén. de Thérapeutique. Nov.

1909   Koch. Munch. Med. Wochenschrift. Avril 17.

1909   J. Piot. Toxicité de l'essence de Mirbane. Parf. Mod. 97.

1909   P. Jucquelier. Action bactéricide des Parfums. Parf. Mod. Mars.

1909   J. Piot. Action de l'Anéthol. Parf. Moderne 13.

1910   H. Kraemer. A Textbook of botany & pharmacognosy. 3° ed.

1910   Martindale. Pharmaceutical Journal et P. E. O. R. Nov.

1910   E. Forgues. Essences déterpénées en chirurgie. Parf. Mod. 36.

1910   E. Forgues. Essences déterpénées en thérapeutiques interne. Parf. Mod. 133.

1910   Classement des essences. Pouvoir antiseptique. Pharmac. Journal II. 609.

1910   P. Jucquelier. Parfums sédatifs. Parf. Moderne 17.

1910   Liotard. Action de certains parfums. Parf. Mod. 103.

1911   Vidal. L'embaumement. Parf. Mod. Janvier 5.

1911   Vendax. Les Parfums et la voix. Parf. Mod. 81.

1911   E. Forgues. Les Parfums en pathologie. Parf. Mod. 106.

1911   Lucas. Preservative materials used by the ancient Egyptian in embalming. Le Caire.

1912   Trillat. La théorie miasmique et les idées du jour. Revue scientifique.

1912   Blaizot et Caldagne. Pouvoir bactéricide de certaines essences. Parf. Mod. 108.

1912   Couetoux de Blain. Le traitement de la phtysie par inhalations. Doin. Paris.

1912   Rochaix. Lois et théories de l'action germicide des substances cliniques. Rev. d'Hyg. et police sanitaire.

1912   Cartaz. Pansements antiseptiques parfumés. La Nature et Parf. Mod. 46.

1912   E. Forgues. Les essences déterpénées contre la dyphtérie. Parf. Mod.

1912   Trillat et Fonassier. C. R. Acad des Sciences.

1913   Guislain G. et Guy Laroche. Bull. Soc. de Biol.

1913   Holmes. F. M. Sur les huiles d'eucalyptus. Pharmac. Journal.

1913   Vaudremer. Action de l'extrait d'aspergiline sur les bacilles. Soc. Biol.

1913   Cabanès. Remèdes d'autrefois. Maloine. Paris.

1913   G. Renaudet. Emploi des huiles essentielles dans le traitement de la phtiriase. Parf. Mod.

1913   David I. Macht. Baltimore. J. Pharmacol. 4.547. Action emménagogue des essences.

1913   R. Geinitz. Influence antiseptique et narcotique des huiles essentielles. Sitzb. Abhand. Rostock. 4.66.

1913   E. Forgues. Les essences dans la Pharmacopée. Parf. Mod.

1914   Orusert. Traitement de l'anchylostomiase par le thymol, l'eucalyptus. Arch. Schiffs u. Tropen Hyg. 17.765.82.

1914   G. Antoine. Purification des vaccins au moyen de l'essence de girofle. Bull. Acad. Roy. méd. Belge. 27 984.95.

1915   Delbet. La Cytophylaxie. Presse médicale Sept. 27.

1915   Trendelenburg. Arch. f. exptl. Path. 79. 154.

1915   Salant et Nelson M. Motter. Memoir in digest of comments in the pharmacopoeia in U.S.A. 339.

1915   Mencière. Réunion médico-chirurgicale de 11º armée, 18 août.

1916   E. Forgues. L'essence déterpénée de lavande contre les plaies de mauvaise nature. Parf. Mod. février.

1916   Cairre. De la valeur et de l'emploi des antiseptiques pour le traitement des plaies de guerre. Thèse Bordeaux.

1916   Chauvin. La France doit préparer elle-même les produits pharmaceutiques. Thèse. Lyon.

1916   Lejars. Eloge de Just. Lucas Championniére. Soc. de Chir. 19 Juillet.

1916   Hartmann. Au sujet de certaines lois de cicatrisation des plaies.

1916   Policard et Philip. Les premiers stades de l'évolution des plaies dans les blessures par éclats d'obus. Lyon chirurgical.

1916   Doyen et Yamanouchi. La flore bactérienne et le traitement des plaies de guerre. Lyon Chirurg.

1916   Leriche. De l'asepsie pure et des moyens physiques dans le traitement des plaies de guerre. Mars. Soc. de Biol.

1916   Naoso Yoshida. Sur l'action antiseptique de l'essence de Cryptomeria Japonica. J. Pharm. Soc. Japan. 413–571.

1916   Fiessinger et Loutaz. Contribution à l'étude des exudats des plais de guerre. Soc. de Biol.

1917   E. Forgues. L'essence déterpénée de lavande contre les plaies anfractueuses. Parf. Mod. Janv.

1917   Reutter de Rosemont. Comment nos pères conservaient leur corps.

1917   Gattefossé et Lamotte. Culture et Industrie des plantes aromatiques. Lyon.

1918   Caneot. Etat actuel des antiseptiques. C. R. Soc. de Biol.

1918   Raphël Dubois. Du rôle de l'olfaction dans les phénomènes de conservation de l'espèce.

1918   E. Demachy. L'odorat chez les insectes.

1918   Lucien Clavel. Valeur antiseptique de certaines huiles essentielles. C. R. Acad. Sciences. 166. 827

1918   D. McMaster. Pouvoir bactéricide des huiles essentielles. Philadephia. J. Inf. Dis. 24. 378.

1919   I. R. Greig Smith. Proc. Leimean. Soc. of New S.W. 44. 72.

1919   Bonnaure. F. Essai sur les propriétés bactéricides de quelques huiles essentielles. Thèse Lyon.

1919   Audibert et Fouquet. Presse Médicale 26. 8 mai.

1919   Guido Cusmando. Gazz. Chim. Italiana. 49.228.

1919   P. Meurisse. Thérapeutique par les huiles essentielles. Perroux. Mâcon.

1919   R. I. Baker et Smith. Med. J. Australia. 2.401.

1919   Floriane. Emplois du Musc Naturel. Parf. Mod.

1919   Lynn. J. Amer. Pharm. Assoc. 8; 103.

1919   J. Gattefossé et Meunissier. Fleurs et Parfums en Chine. Parf. Mod. Sept.

1919   Volpino. Etude expérimentale sur la thérapie de la tuberculose. Ann. Inst. Pasteur, 3 Mars.

1919   R. M. Gattefossé. Propriétés bactéricides de quelques huiles essentielles. Parf. Mod. 152.

1919   E. Forgues. Le Salvol dans quelques applications nouvelles. Parf. Mod. 34.

1920   Xavier Faucillon. Essence de Cyprès. Parf. Mod. 67.

1920   Gunn. J. Pharm. and Exptol. Therap. 16. 39.

1920   I. R. Greig Smith. Pouvoir germicide de l'essence d'eucalyptus. Soc. of N.S.W. 44. 311.

1920   G. S. Stokvis. Pouvoir bactéricide des vapeurs d'essences. Cent. Bakl. Parasitenk. Abt. I. Amsterdam 85. 165.

1920   J. W. C. Guim. Action carminative des huiles essentielles. Univ. Coll. J. Pharmacol. 16. 39.

1920   L. Giraud. Le lavandin et son essence. Pouvoir bactéricide. Thèse Lyon.

1920   J. Gattefossé. Les ressources aromatiques du Maroc. Parf. Mod. Oct.

1920   Durrans. Perfumery record. 11.391.

1920   J. Balvay. Injections trachéales et tuberculose pulmonaire. Lyon.

1920   P. Meurisse. Asepsie et antisepsie. Parf. Mod. 68.

1921   F. Marre. Les parfums qui font dormir. Parf. Mod.

1921   Penfold et Grant. Proc. Linnaeàn Soc. N.S.W. 58.117.

1921   Morel et Rochaix. C. R. Soc. de Biol. 7 Novembre.

1921   Massy R. Goudron marocain de cedrus atlanticus. Journ de Pharm. et de Chimie. 34. 294.

1921   Massy R. Sur l'essence de cèdre marocain. B. Soc. Sc. Nat. du Maroc. 1.152.

1921   R. Lautier. L'essence de cèdre dans le traitement de la blennorragie aiguë et chronique. Bull. Soc. de Ther. 227.

1921   R. Huerre. L'essence d'oxycèdre, succédané de l'ess. de santal. Bull. Soc. de Thér. 26.126; et essence de cèdre et blennorragie, même bulletin 251.

1921   A. Rolet. Le thymol antelmintique. Parf. Mod. 222.

1921   Cori et Cori. Therap. Halbmonats 36.256.

1921   D. I. Macht et W. M. Kumkel. Action antiseptique de quelques fumées aromatiques. Proc. Soc. Exptl. Biol. Med. 18.68.

1921   D. I. Macht et Gin Ching Ting. Propriétés sédatives de quelques drogues aromatiques et fumées. J. Pharmacol. 18.361.

1921   A. D. Hirschelder et L. J. Pankow. L'introduction d'un groupe ethoxy dans les composés aromatiques augmente-t-elle l'action bactéricide sur le pneumocoque et le gonocoque. Soc. Exptl. Biol. Méd. 19; 64.

1922   G. Gatti et Cayola. Action thérapeutique des huiles essentielles. Rev. Ital. Ess. Prof. 4; 16 et 4; 77.

1922   Morel et Rochaix. C. R. Soc. Biol. Mai.

1922   Penfold et Grant. Proc. Linnaen Soc. N.S.W. 44.311.

1922   Trabut. L. Le Libanol. Rev. Horticole de l'Algérie. 72.

1922   Delange. Rev. Scien. 60.505.

1922   J. Marchand. Observations relatives à des affections vénériennes traitées par la lavande. Parf. Mod. 189.

1922   Lestrat. Le juniperus Phœnica. Thèse.

1922   De Beaupré J. Les derniers cèdres du Liban. Parf. Mod. 123.

1922   G. Gatti et Cayola. Action thérapeutique des huiles essentielles. Parf. Mod. 227.

1922   Lepinay et R. Massy. Essai d'application en dermatologie du goudron et de l'essence de cèdre de l'Atlas. Bull. Soc. Franc. de dermatologie et Syphil. 35.

1922   Velu. Antiseptie par les essences en médecine vétérinaire. Parf. Mod. 133.

1922   J. Gattefossé. Les plantes aromatiques dans la thérapeutique indigène au Maroc. Parf. Mod. 110.

1922   A. Sassard. Le genre Hyssopus et Satureia. Thèse. Toulouse.

1922   Alexander. Lancet. 25 mars 605.

1922   Dubosc A. Le Camphre et sa synthèse. Lyon.

1922   Riv. Ital. delle ess. e Profumi 4.96 et 4.127.

1922   Trabut L. Culture industrielle du Camphrier. Lyon.

1922   Raynaud L. Essence de cèdre et blennorragie. Maroc. Med. 15 Mai.

1922   Evrard. L'essence de cèdre dans le traitement de la blennorragie. Maroc. Med. 15 février.

1922   F. A. Millet. J. Soc. Chem. Industry. 41.467.

1923   R. Massy. Contribution à l'étude des produits susceptibles d'être fournis par les forêts du Maroc. Bull. Soc. Sc. Nat. du Maroc. 25.111.

1923   A. F. Morgan. La vitamine A dans quelques essences d'Hespéridées. Am. J. physiol. 64.522.

1923   O. H. Pant et G. H. Miller. Effets carminatifs des huiles essentielles. J. Pharmacol. 21. Proc. 203.

1923   A. R. Penfold et R. Grant. J. Proc. Roy. Soc. N.S.W. 56.219.

1923   G. Alfonso. Action thérapeutique des essence d'amandes amères et de menthe. Rev. Ital. ess. prof. 4. 4.

1923   Correlation between chemical constitution and therapeutic value. Ind. J. Medicine 11.337.

1923   Stevens. A textbook of therapeutics 6° ed. Londres.

1923   Pic et Bonnamour. Phytothérapie et médicaments végétaux. Paris.

1923   J. Gattefossé. Parfums berbères. Le Tauserghimt. Parf. Mod. Juin.

1923   G. Petit. Parfums et remèdes tirés des gastéropodes. Parf. Mod. 57.

1923   E. Tant. L'essence de cèdre dans le traitement de la blennorragie. Bruxelles Médical. 20 décembre.

1923   Penfold et Grant. Valeur germicide des principales ess. d'eucalyptus. J. Proc. Roy. Soc. N.S.W. 57.80, 58.117, 57.211.

1923   J. C. Delage. Emploi de l'essence de moutarde en œnologie. Ann. Fals. 16.483.

1924   G. Gatti et Cayola. Emploi des huiles essentielles contre la chute des cheveux. Rev. Ital. ess. Prof. 5.85.

1924   J. Alt. Wegg. U.S. 1.483 feb. 12. Emplois du thym et girofle mélangés à de la bile comme produit pharmaceutique.

1924   Otto Schôbb. Comparison du pouvoir antiseptique du Chaulmogra avec les autres essences. Philippine J. Soc. 24.23.

1924   Otto Schôbb et Hirosch Kusama. Pouvoir désinfectant des vapeurs organiques. Philippine J. Scien. 24.443.

1924   K. N. Chopra et Premankur. Action thérapeutique de l'es. de Kuth Saussurea Lappa. India Med. Gaz. 59.540.

1924   Smillie and Pessoa. J. Pharmacol. 24.359.

1924   R. M. Gattefossé et J. Tamisier. Considérations sur l'action antitoxique des huiles essentielles. IVe Congrès pour l'avancement des Sciences. Liège.

1924   Siegel. Arch. f. exptl. Pharm. u. Patho. 104.323.

1924   R. M. Gattefossé et Tamisier. Rôle physiologique des Parfums. Legendre Lyon.

1924   V. Braun et Cochin. Berichte 57. B. 373.

1924   R. M. Gattefossé. Relations entre les fonctions chimiques et les propriétés physiologiques des corps odorants. Chimie et Industrie. Mai.

1924   Fraevenitz Arch. Fur exptl. Path. U. Pharm. 104 289.

1924   C. V. A. Duffaut. De l'essence de cèdre en thérapeutique. Thèse. Bordeaux.

1924   Bryant. P.E.O.R. Déc.

1924   Cl. Roux. Produits odorants d'origine animale. Lyon.

1924   Dyche Teague. P.E.O.R. Janvier. Février, Mars.

1924   A. J. Van Laren. On the culture of chenopodium. Pharm Weekblad n° 22.

1924   H. Leclerc. Le cédre de l'Atlas. Presse méd. 16 août.

1924   Hogstadt. Amer. Journal of Pharmacy. 96.809.

1924   Dorat, Massy et Marquis. Sur un extrait pyroligneux de thuya et son aplication en médecine vétérinaire. Bull des sciences Nat. du Maroc. 214.

1924   J. Bryant. Valeur détergente et antiseptique des huiles ess. P.E.O.R. 15.426.

1925   F. Ch. Et. Roux. Le Calycanthus occidentalis et son essence. Thèse. Lyon.

1925   H. A. Gardner. Effets physiologiques des vapeurs de solvants. Paint. Manuf. Assoc. of V.S. circ. n° 250 89.149.

1925   A. Morel et Rochaix. Société de Biol. 7 Novemb.

1925   Mayers et Thienes. J. Amer. Med. Assoc. 84. 1895. Pouvoir fongicide de certaines essences.

1925   Karwacki et Biernacki. Ann. Inst. Pasteur XXXIX. 476.

1925 C. Reynolds. The Industrial Chemist. Février.

1925 R. M. Gattefossé et Douly. Action physiologique des solutions aromatiques. Chimie et Industrie. Septembre.

1925 Nazzareno Grisogani. Relations entre le rythme de la sécrétion paratidique et les sensations olfactives et gustatives de l'homme. Atti. acad. Lincei. 1.602. 4.

1925 V. Niclot. Une gloire thérapeutique ancienne, le cèdre. Progrès médical 13-12-24 et Maroc Médical 15 avril 1925.

1925 Louis Fondard et Ernest Autran. Menthe et lavande. Parfums de France n° 23.

1925 Otto Schôbb. Effets antiseptiques des vapeurs des huiles essentielles. Philippine J. Scien. 26.501.

1925 Penfold et Grant. Pouvoir germicide de quelques essences australiennes et de leurs constituants. J. Proc. Roy. Soc. N.S.W. 59.346.

1925 Bogert. American Perfumer 20.453.

1926 R. Massy. Etude analytique des goudrons de conifère. Bordeaux.

1926 Kuns Krause. Publication in honour of Tschirch's jubilee. Leipzig.

1926 La pharmacopée norvégienne et les huiles essentielles. Bull. Fédér. Pharmaciens du S.O. et Centre.

1926 H. Leclerc. La Tanaisie. Presse Médicale 1437. 13.11.

1926 Les huiles essentielles dans la pharmacopée allemande. Bull. Féd. Pharmaciens du S.O. et Centre.

1926 R. M. Gattefossé. Valeur thérapeutique de l'essence de lavande. Parf. Mod. 152.

1926 J. Marchand. Observations relatives à des cas d'infection vénérienne. Parf. Mod. 154.

1926 R. M. Gattefossé. Les essences en thérapeutique. Parf. Mod. 229.

1926 Myers. J. Pharmacol. 27.248.

1926 J. J. Bryant. P.E.O.R. et Chem. Zeitung.

1926 Penfold et Grant. Proc. Linnaen Soc. N.S.W. 60.167. Valeur germicide de quelques essences australiennes.

1926 T. Kuroda. Influence de la concentration des ions H sur l'action antiseptique de quelques phénols et composés aromatiques. Biochem. Z. 169. 281.

1926 J. W. Tomb. Prévention et traitement du choléra par les huiles essentielles. J. Trop. Med. Hyg. 29.210.

1926 W. Wiechowski. Les huiles essentielles en médecine. Karlsbader aerztl. Vôrtrâge 7.484.531.

1926 Plant et Miller. J. Pharmacol. 26.149.

1926 Da Costa. C. R. Soc. Biol. 95.1273.

1926 Joachimoglu. Deutsche Mediz. Wochensch. 49. 2079.

1926 Flury et Steel. Munchener Médiz. Wochensch. 73.20.

1926 Cerbelaud. Parfumerie Mod. 19.3.13.

1927 R. M. Gattefossé. Cicatrisation rapide des plaes par les huiles essentielles. Parf. Mod. 12.

1927   G. Renaudet. Propriétés et emplois thérapeutiques des parfums. Parfumerie Mod. Nov.

1927   Empiriques d'autrefois. Chronique médicale n° 70.

1927   P. Courmont. A. Morel et I. Bay. C. R. Soc. Biol. XCVI, 1313.

1927   S. G. Willomott et Frank Wokes. Vitamines contenues dans les essences de citron. P.E.O.R. 18.257.

1927   Kenzo Tamura Hideo Uchida et Gyokroy Kihara. Action du camphre du Japon sur le cœur. Proc. Imp. Acad. Japan 3.557.70.

1927   Léon et Henri Buret. Etude biologique des injections. J. Phar. Chim. 6.288.

1927   J. M. Schaeffer & F. W. Tilley. Relations entre la constitution chimique et le pouvoir germicide des alcools et phénols. J. Bact. 14.259.

1927   Berlingozzi. Gazzetta Chimica Italiana 57.264.

1927   Christomanos. Klinische Wochensch. 39.1859.

1927   Dyson et Hunter. J. Chem. Soc. 1186.

1927   Bogert. Americ. Perfumer. 22.63.

1927   A. Morel et Rochaix. C. R. Soc. de Biol. XCVI. 1311. Mai.

1928   Dyson. Chemistry by chemotherapy. Benn.

1928   Tamendo O. Kaniski. Action pharmacologique du santal des aiguilles de pin et du vétyver. Fol. Pharm. Jap. 7.77.

1928   J. Ferrua. Physiologie des hormones végétales. Parf.-Mod. 59.

1928   Dyson. Perfumery Record. 19 3.88.171 341.

1928   H. Leclerc. Emploi de l'essence de sassafras comme antispasmodique. Presse Médicale, p. 700. 2 Juin.

1928   Morel, Rochaix et Sevelinge. R. Soc. de Biol. XCVIII. 47.

1928   H. Leclerc. Propriétés antispasmodiques, antiseptiques, parasiticides et diurétiques de la lavande. Presse Médicale, p. 1133–1134. Sept. 5.

1928   Rideal Rideal et Sciver. P.E.O.R. Special number 290.

1928   Ellery H. Harvey. Les huiles essentielles comme antienzymes. Am. J. Pharma. 100–524.

1928   L. B. Kingery et A. Adkisson. Emploi d'huiles essentielles comme fungicides. Arch. Dermatol. Syphil. 17.499.

1929   Rideal S. R. Action germicide de certaines essences. Parf. Mod. 61.

1929   J. Ferrua. Action physiologique des essences sur les centres nerveux. Parf. Mod. 341.

1929   S. Malowan. Utilisation pharmacologique des parfums synthétiques. Riechstoffindustrie 4.90.

1929   Stanley. G. Willimott. Vitamines et autres produits dans les essences de citron. P.E.O.R. 20.270.

1929   Walter. Action antiseptique des huiles essentielles. Riechstoffindustrie 4.12.

1929   George F. Reddish. Méthode de dosage du pouvoir antiseptique. J. Lab. Clin. Med. 14.649.

1930 Dyson. Aspects physiologiques des huiles essentielles. P.E.O.R. Londres 287.

1930 A. Morel et Rochaix C. R. Soc. Biol. 19 Mai et 20 Juin.

1930 Malcolm Dyson. Physiological aspect of ess. oils. P.E.O.R. 21.

1930 F. Pasteur. Sur la fenchone. Union. pharm. N° 6. 71ᵉ V.

1930 Coulthard Marshall et Pymann. Journ. Chem. Soc. 280.

1930 M. Renaud. Les savons en thérapeutique. Rev. Crit. de path. et thérapeutique.

1930 Ruth et Miller. Institut de recherche de Philadelphie. C. R.

1930 Arno Müller. Riechstoffindust 5.102 4.126.8. Nouvelle méthode physique pour le test des huiles essentielles.

1930 Vincent et Velluz. C. R. Acad. des sciences. 16 Mars.

1930 R. Naves. L'essence de lavande en pharmacie. Parfums de France. Sept. 259.

1930 H. Leclerc. Histoire du romarin. Janus 196. Juillet.

1930 Vincent. C. R. Académie des Sciences. 22 Sept.

1930 C. Phillip. Préparation de nouveaux désinfectants à base de thymol et de carvacrol. Arch. Hyg. 105.15.

1930 Ph. Kuhn. Action des désinfectants à base de thymol et de carvacrol. Arch. Hyg. 18.28.

1930 Eric. K. Rideal. A. Sciver et N. E. G. Richardson. Pouvoir germicide et activité capillaire de certaines huiles essentielles. P.E.O.R. 21.341.

1930 W. A. Collier et Y. Nitta. Action d'huiles essentielles contenant des éthers sur certaines bactéries. Z. Hyg. Infektionkrankh. 111.

1930 Tatsumi Nagira et Taro Yao. Les agents employés contre le mal de dents. Folia Pharmacol. Japan 9. N° 4.

1930 P. K. De. Etude de la désinfection et de la stérilisation. De India J. Med. Research. 18.83.

1930 P. K. De et Subrahmanyan. Propriétés germicides de certaines huiles essentielles indoues. India. J. Med. research 17.1153.

1931 Siegfried L. Malowam. Action germicide des essences éthérés. Z. Hyg. Infektionkrankh 112.93.

1931 F. U. Rapp. Quelques emplois de l'ess. de pin. Insec. Desinf. 7. N° 9 93; 113. 115.

1931 C. Philipp et P. H. Kuhn. Production du thymol et du carvacrol. Pharm. Press. Wiss. Prekt. Heft. 19.

1931 Ruth. E. Miller. Activité bactéricide des huiles essentielles. Am. J. Pharm. 103 324.

1931 W. Morrel Roberts Quart. Effets des Huiles essentielles sur la sécrétion gastrique. J. Med. 24.133.

1931 J. Boucher. Soc. de Therap. 10 décembre.

1931 M. Renaud. Les savons en thérapeutique. Janv. et fév. Revue Crit. de Path. et Thérap.

1931 P. Sassard. Traitement des plaies atones par l'essence de lavande. Parfumerie Moderne 395.

1931   L. Sevelinge. Pouvoir bactéricide du menthol. Parfum. Mod. Mars et avril.

1931   Irvine W. Humphrey. Emplois des produits du pin. Trans. Inst. Chem. Engrs London 9.40.

1931   H. Leclerc. Action cholagogue du romarin. Press. Med. Janvier p. 124.

1932   Ch. Ranaivo. Sur le Rambiazina. Parf. Mod. 491.

1932   E. R. Miller. Efficacité bactéricide des huiles essentielles. Parf. Mod. 105.

1932   R. M. Gattefossé. Usi terapeutici dell'essenza di bergamotto. Rome.

1932   G. Genin. Emploi des huiles essentielles comme bactéricides. Parf. Mod. 87.

1932   R. M. Gattefossé. Emplois thérapeutiques de l'essence de lavande. Parf. Mod. 533.

1932   R. M. Gattefossé. La lavande en thérapeutique. Parf. Mod. 441.

1932   Pierre Sassard. Essai de synthèse sur les propriétés et applications thérapeutiques du Sapolinol. Bull. Méd. Févr 32.

1932   R. M. Gattefossé. L'essence de pin et ses propriétés bactéricides. Parf. Mod. 559.

1932   Y. R. Naves. Vitamines et terpènes. Parfums de France. Avril.

1932   P. Sassard. Le traitement des plaies. Parfum. Mod. 239.

1932   Micheli Mitolo. Action inhibitrice d'huiles essentielles sur les microorganismes. Boll. Soc. Ital. Biol. Sper. 7.220.

1932   C. Forti. Action de certaines substances volatiles sur les leucocytes en vie. Boll. Soc. Ital. Biol. Sper. 7.234.

1932   H. Leclerc. L'hydrolat de fleur d'oranger. Presse Méd. p. 1328. 27 août.

1932   R. R. Read et Ellis Miller. Quelques substituts du phénol et leur activité germicide. J. Am. Chem. Soc. 54.1195.

1932   T. Gordonoff et F. Janett. Thym et thymol comme expectorants et désinfectants pour la langue. Z. Ges. Expte. med. 79.486.

1932   A. R. Penfold. Plantes australiennes antiseptiques. J. Chem. education 9.428.

1932   Frank Wokes. Toxicité des isomères du menthol. Quart J. Pharm. 5.233.

1933   Katleen Culhane et S. W. F. Underhill. Chemist & Druggist. Fév.

1933   Pont. Dentifrices et la Flore Buccale. Parf. Mod. Fév.

1933   R. M. Gattefossé. Le Pouvoir antiseptique du terpophène. Parf. Mod. Mai.

BIOGRAPHY

RENÉ-MAURICE GATTEFOSSÉ

1881–1950

From the end of his studies, R.-M. Gattefossé showed a real taste for invention: chemical and photographic equipment, new pneumatic tyres and new elastic materials, reaction motor, application of acetylene etc. However his father, Louis Gattefossé, showed him that his brilliant imaginative capacity could be most fruitfully applied to perfumery if he devoted himself exclusively to this area.

Louis Gattefossé, at this time and indeed since the international exhibition of Lyon (1894), had added to the business which he managed with his elder son, Abel, the import of exotic essential oils and the export of synthetic perfumes. The chemistry of perfumes in the region of Lyon was then in its early days.

Synthetic perfumes, mixtures of natural essential oils, alcoholic extracts, *enfleurage* ointments and synthetic products had not even reached a rudimentary level. None of the fragrant products available to perfumers had the same power. Some were greatly diluted in alcohol (*lavage* ointments), others high in terpenes (essential oils) and the synthetic perfumes themselves were sold diluted and at ill-defined concentrations.

In close collaboration, Louis, Abel and René-Maurice Gattefossé endeavoured to determine the conditions under which it would be possible to prepare compositions of a constant strength and smell and succeeded firstly in preparing concentrated products and soon 100% perfumes as they are prepared today.

As these new products had to be used very differently from normal trade items, perfumers had to be instructed as to their use and this was the origin of the first Gattefossé perfumery formulary (1906), with subsequent reprints reaching record figures.

1906 to 1912 was a boom time for new methods of formulation, those which enabled French perfumes to be prepared as they are today. Synthetic creations multiplied, terpeneless essences, invented by Haensel from Pirna (Czechoslovakia), enabled compositions to be obtained which were more constant and more soluble than natural essential oils. Finally, the industry in Grasse produced absolute essences of flowers which was the finishing touch to modern formulation.

In 1908, M. de Fontgalland, president of the Agricultural Trade Union Association in the South-West, informed the Gattefossés of the misery of lavender growers in the mountainous regions of

Drome, Vaucluse and the Lower Alps. This was the start of the "La Parfumerie Moderne" campaign, created for this purpose to increase the value of lavender essence and later for its rational distillation and its cultivation.

These unexpected developments in the lavender industry produced, in just a few years, a marked prosperity in what had hitherto been the most underprivileged areas of France – in the *départements* where seasonal or definitive emigration was a custom and where villages were being depopulated.

R.-M. Gattefossé thus helped M. Mus in his organisation for the cultivation of mint in France, an area which had been abandoned due to the competition from English mint. He also introduced from Italy the cultivation of clary sage, used in Italy in the preparation of vermouth, but which he distilled for the first time to obtain one of the most remarkable essences in the composer's laboratory. Finally, he undertook the systematic study of exotic essential oils, defined and described types of stills which were easy to make in the bush and, thanks to his encouragement, numerous French colonies undertook this industry or developed it.

The war of 1914 to 1918 disorganised the Maison Gattefossé, the founder of which, Louis Gattefossé, died in 1910. As Abel and Robert Gattefossé died for their country, René-Maurice Gattefossé was aided by his young brother, Jean Gattefossé.

In order to continue his study of colonial products, René-Maurice sent Jean, a botanist and chemist, to Morocco, following the very trail of the army of pacification. This journey to Morocco enabled a large number of new plants to be catalogued and a flourishing distillation industry to be organised in the protectorate. All these works at the time were published in the magazine *Parfumerie Moderne*.

Numerous applications of essential oils made by peasants and natives as popular remedies had attracted R-M Gattefossé's attention and he sought to find out the causes and verify their efficacity. After having had the opportunity to check the extraordinary merits on himself following a laboratory explosion, he devoted most of his time to this area of study. After an initial work published under the name of Dr Meurisse, on products prepared specially, venereology tests by Dr Marchand, colonial applications of the senior medical officer Forgues, the veterinary surgeon Velu, he published with Dr Tamisier: *Considérations sur l'emploi des huiles essentielles* [Reflections on the use of essential oils] (IV Congress for the advancement of science, Liège 1923), then *Rôle physiologique des parfums*

[Physiological role of perfumes] (1924) with Doully, *Action physiologique des solutions aromatiques* [Physiological action of aromatic solutions] (4th Chemical Congress), and in Roma *Usi Terapeutici dell'essenze di Bergamotta* [Therapeutic uses of Bergamot essence], an award-winning work in Italy.

Finally, in 1937 his two main works appeared: *Aromathérapie* [Aromatherapy] and *Antiseptiques essentieles* [Essential antiseptics], which have since had profound repercussions on the use of these products.

His works in this field did not however stop, thanks to the welcome offered him by certain hospitals in Lyon, where he was able to continue his tests with the help of a number of doctors.

It was moreover by the application of aromatics in dermatology that he launched the works of his colleagues in this field. Thanks to research carried out in his laboratory, the technique of harmless or therapeutic beauty products made enormous progress. Well known works have popularised these concepts: *Produits de Beauté* [Beauty Products] (1936), translated into Spanish, Italian and Polish, and *Esthétique physiologique* [Physiological aesthetics] (1938) etc.

These are the principal professional works of R-M Gattefossé, but an activity such as this could not be confined to industrial research. His main interests were pre-history and metaphysics and in these subjects he published works remarkable for their daring. They are: *Volonté et force psychique* [Will and psychic force], *L'Ame inconnue de la Patrie* [The unknown soul of the mother country], *Adam, homme tertiaire* [Adam, tertiary man], *La vérité sur l'Atlantide* [The truth of Atlantis], *Les origines préhistoriques de l'Ecriture* [The pre-historic origins of writing], *Un conflit européen a l'époque néolithique* [A European conflict in the Neolithic age], *Le roman de Marthe la Salyenne* [The story of Marthe la Salyenne], *Les Sages Ecritures* [The Wise Writings].

There were also some local history essays: *Images de Lyon* [Images of Lyon], and *A l'Ombre du Clocher* [In the shadow of the Clock Tower], a science fiction novel: *Paradis S.A.*, and because of his collaboration with scientific reviews, quantities of notes and miscellaneous articles.

This is, in brief, the product of the career of a man devoted to the service of a profession, for he paid great service to the French perfumery industry, the pleasant economy in the mountains, and French colonies, services which were reflected by a major increase in export and by a world-wide reputation for the technical quality of French laboratories. Thirty-three works of great originality and 42 years at the head of an influential international journal did not prevent R-M Gattefossé from running the family business prudently and devoting all his leisure time to collective interests, as secretary, and later as vice-president, of the Lyon Perfumerie Syndicate, group leader at the Lyon Trade Fair and founder of the A.I.C.A.

Tirelessly, he inspired those around him to question all contemporary knowledge with a view to adapting it to the techniques and new lifestyle which was inevitably to follow the Second World War.

THE WORKS OF R-M GATTEFOSSÉ

Chemistry of perfume and cosmetics:

1906 Formulaire de Parfumerie (3 éditions).

1908 Création de la revue de défense professionnelle «La Parfumerie Moderne».

1916 Lavande et Spic (en collaboration avec M. Lamothe). Culture et industrie des plantes aromatiques.

1919 Technique de la Fabrication des Parfums.

1923 Considération sur l'emploi des huiles essentielles (en collaboration avec D. Tamisier).

1923 Formulary of the parisian perfumer.

1924 Rôle physiologique des parfums (en collaboration avec D. Tamisier).

1925 Action physiologique des solutions aromatiques (avec M. Douly).

1926 Distillation des plantes aromatiques et des parfums.

1926 Nouveaux parfums de synthèse (en collaboration avec Jean Gattefossé) (2 éditions).

1927 Agenda du chimiste parfumeur (2 éditions).

1932 Usi terapeutici dell'essenza di bergamotta (Rome).

1936 Produits de beauté.

1937 Aromathérapie.

1937 Antiseptiques essentiels.

1937 Productos de belleza, traduction espagnole de Produits de Beauté.

1938 Cosmetica moderna (traduction italienne de Produits de Beauté).

1938 Esthétique physiologique.

1939 Produkty kosmetyczne (traduction polonaise de Produits de Beauté).

1940 Essai de bio-physique (en collaboration avec Dr H. Jonquières).

1941   Contribution à l'étude physico-chimique de la peau (en collaboration avec Dr H. Jonquières, Dr P. Cuilleret, E. Mahler, H. M. Gattefossé).

1945   Technique des Produits de Beauté (en collaboration avec le Dr H. Jonquières) (traduction en langue anglaise).

1947   Théorie de la chevelure (en collaboration avec le Dr H. Jonquières).

1949   Formulaire de parfumerie et cosmétologie (traduction en langue anglaise).

Archeology – Prehistory – Philosophy:

1911   Volonté et force psychique.

1917   L'Ame inconnue de la patrie.

1919   Adam, l'homme tertaire.

1923   La vérité sur l'Atlantide.

1925   Origines préhistoriques de l'écriture.

1927   Un conflit européen à l'époque néolithique.

1934   Métaphysique préhistorique.

1940   Paradis, société anonyme.

1942   Le roman de Marthe la Salyenne.

1945   Les Sages écritures.

1948   La République des Anges

En collaboration avec Germaine Piroird:

1935   Images de Lyon (2 volumes).

1937   A l'ombre du clocher.

NOTES

PREFACE

1. Thymol is extracted from essential oil of thyme, and is its major constituent.

FOREWORD

2. A perceptive observation. The impurities referred to here, found in synthetic reproductions of natural compounds, do indeed alter their properties.

3. This is a misunderstanding by the author. Not all plants are fragrant, and not all plants contain an essential oil. Approximately 25% of medicinal herbs are aromatic.

4. The scientific study of essential oils is currently addressing both of these questions.

5. Essential oils have little or nothing in common with vitamins (which at that time had recently been discovered).

6. Essential oils have very few known functions in plants, and certainly have little in common with animal hormones. They are not indispensable to plant life in general.

CHAPTER I

7. We now know that a great many insects use odours as signals. Many of these odours are identical with chemicals found in essential oils.

8. These animal secretions are no longer included as substances used in aromatherapy.

9. Not all plants contain essential oils.

10. Aromatic plants are those which contain essential oil. Non-aromatic plants contain no essential oil.

11. These are now commonly known as "absolutes".

12. Citrus oils are sometimes distilled today, but the expressed oils are widely and safely used in food flavours and in aromatherapy.

13. This is an ambitious statement. We now know that plants do contain hormones but these are not the essential oils. Also see note 6.

CHAPTER II

14. Gattefossé's dislike of terpenes is unfounded in the light of recent toxicology data, and his preference for terpeneless essential oils is shared by very few aromatherapists today. Terpeneless oils, although obtainable, are relatively costly and very different from the whole, natural oil.

15. Since thymol and carvacrol are the components which lend irritancy and some toxicity to thyme oil, terpeneless thyme will be more, not less hazardous, than the natural oil.

CHAPTER III

16. The oil of roses mentioned in the literature is sometimes rose essential oil, but more often it is an infused oil, made by heating a mixture of new petals and fatty oil.

17. Bdellium is a gum similar to myrrh. Ancient literature often confuses the two, and it is likely that Lemery was here referring to myrrh itself.

18. Kills tapeworm.

19. It is curious that Gattefossé makes no allusion here to asafoetida's most celebrated feature – its unpleasant odour!

20. This is an exaggeration. Any strong odour has the potential to cause headache, if inhaled for long enough and possibly migraines in those prone to them.

CHAPTER IV

22. Some essential oils do have a mild anaesthetic property.

23. This statement is incorrect. For example:
(Wood Oils)	Rosewood oil has 2% terpenes
	Sandalwood has 2% terpenes
(Leaf Oils)	Peppermint has 10% terpenes
	Melissa has 10% terpenes.
(Flower Oils)	Neroli has 15% terpenes
	Ylang Ylang has 25% terpenes

24. All essential oils are inflammable, about as much as alcohol or paraffin.

25. Eucalyptol, or cineole, is the main chemical component of eucalyptus oil, and is usually found at around 75%.

26. Revulsive means counter-irritant, i.e. producing or diverting irritation.

27. Terpenes are indeed very useful for dissolving mucus. However, they do not cause the problems that the author lists here unless, perhaps, if taken in abnormally high doses.

28. Most essences are not regarded as caustic or toxic today, and removing terpenes will not necessary make them safer in any way.

29. Eucalyptol (cineole) is now known to possess antibacterial and expectorant properties.

30. Eucalyptus, like several other essential oils, can be bought "crude", containing some dissolved water from the distillation process, or "dehydrated", with the water removed.

31. The author seems to want the oil to oxidise through light exposure. However, it is now recognised that UV rays cause the production of (harmful) free radicals in most essential oils. For this reason, they should be kept in amber glass bottles.

32. The camphor referred to here is not very highly toxic, although it has some toxicity. The fact of being a ketone does not automatically indicate toxicity, although it is true that many ketones found in essential oils are toxic.

33. Antidote to poison.

34. Camphor is indeed anaphrodisiac (the opposite of aphrodisiac) but again, these generalisations do not hold for all ketones.

35. The author is referring to the equivalent ester of linalol, linalyl acetate.

36. Probably sclareol and sclareol oxide.

37. These spasms are only produced by very high, toxic amounts. Such spasms are more readily produced by ketones than esters.

38. This is equivalent to an adult drinking about 200ml (8oz) of essential oil.

39. Benzyl benzoate is found in oils of Peru balsam, tuberose and ylang-ylang.

40. There are several "artemisia essences" most of which are regarded as toxic and abortifacient due to their thujone content.

41. I know of no evidence that carvone is toxic.

42. Most phenols are indeed caustic, notably thymol, which can severely irritate mucous membrane.

43. The removal of certain essential oil components, whether terpenes or not, may sometimes lead to a more powerful action on one level, but the essential oil is no longer natural. Nevertheless, a few aromatherapists do use terpeneless oils today.

44. Instead of artificially removing toxic components from essential oils the modern trend in aromatherapy is either to avoid using a few oils altogether, or to seek chemotypes which contain only very small quantities of the undesirable components.

45. The author is suggesting that essential oils should not be used with fatty substances, such as vegetable oils. This is certainly not in line with present trends, in which massage using this combination is so popular.

46. Phytol is a component of jasmine absolute.

47. Some essential oils do, of course, present certain dangers. Unlike vitamins essential oils are not, in themselves, nutrients, nor is there any evidence that the body can change them into nutritive substances. Nevertheless, the chemical similarities referred to are interesting.

48. This concept of synergy remains a strong belief in current aromatherapy thinking.

49. Anti-pus i.e. antiseptic.

50. Wound-healing.

51. Drying.

52. Coughing up of blood, often found in people with tuberculosis.

53. Elecampane oil, now known to carry a high risk of causing allergic reaction when applied to the skin. *Inula graveolens*, however, is increasingly used in aromatherapy.

54. Labiate essences include mints, sages, rosemary, lavender, marjoram, melissa and many others.

55. Administering sodium cinnamate by subcutaneous injection may well be effective, but it is a long way from being aromatherapy by today's definitions.

56. The cedar referred to here is *Cedrus atlantica*, or Atlas cedarwood.

57. The disadvantages of oral administration listed here are very debatable, and should not be taken as proven. Gattefossé's opinion is not shared by many French doctors today.

58. The rectal route of administration has many advantages – rapid absorption, no enzyme metabolism – and is frequently used by medical aromatherapists today, especially for respiratory disorders.

59. This is one of Gattefossé's great insights, and it was this vision of dermal administration which led to the modern renaissance of massage/aromatherapy. (It is curious, however, that this method was only suggested for pulmonary disorders.)

60. Percutaneous absorption of essential oils has been fairly well researched over the past 50 years, and is now accepted as proven. Warmth is known to aid absorption, and the removal of excess sebum is also likely to help.

61. Covering the skin after application prevents much evaporation, and greatly enhances absorption.

62. Thymol would perhaps be a "perfect antiseptic" if it was not so irritating.

63. Gattefossé seems to be advocating the administration of pure essential oil to the skin, something rarely done in aromatherapy today. If he did not believe that ointments would permit penetration due to their greasiness, he would probably not advocate the use of vegetable oil as a penetration vehicle.

64. It cannot be said that Gattefossé does not mention massage, albeit fleetingly! This would be more of a "friction rub" than the type of massage given in aromatherapy today.

65. It should be remembered that the medical meaning of narcosis is stupor leading to insensibility, e.g. a general anaesthetic used during surgery.

66. Warming the body by applying mildly irritant oils.

67. Gattefossé's recognition of the psycho-neurological action of essential oils shows his broad vision for aromatherapy.

68. Benzaldehyde is the major component of bitter almond essence.

69. Methyl anthranilate is found in orange flowers.

70. A hypnotic is a substance which induces sleep.

71. Analgesic perhaps, but mildly so.

72. Many factors, including current mood can influence the outcome of testing the effects of essential oils on the psyche, and such experiments are indeed very difficult.

73. The toxic and convulsive effects of thujone are now well documented. It is also found, in quantity, in oils of thuja, mugwort, wormwood and sage.

74. Aids digestion.

75. Rumbling or gurgling made by gas in intestines.

76. Promoting the flow of bile.

77. This type of research may have led to the development of mentholated cigarettes.

78. Again, I have to disagree.

79. These were made by heating a mixture of dried aromatic plants and fatty oil.

80. See note 54.

81. Any type of skin condition where there are flakes or scales resembling bran.

82. Itchy and bumpy.

83. Any type of skin condition where there are flakes or scales resembling bran.

84. A type of bacterium found in gonorrhoea.

85. *Piper matico*, a tree of the piperaceae family which grows in Brazil and Peru. An essential oil is found in the leaves.
    A Non-syphilitic venereal ulceration.
    B Inflamed sore.
    C Rapid ulceration.
    D Tumours.
    E Inflammation of penis.
    F A micro-organism related to syphilis.
    G Vegetable oil which has been chemically treated so that it dissolves in water.
    H Sudden and overwhelming.
    J Phenol, or carbolic acid, was used for its disinfectant power.
    K A test for syphilis.

L 100 or 200 grams (4–8oz) of pure essential oil seems an enormous quantity for a bath!

86. These cases, although the information given is sparse, constitute impressive evidence of the antiseptic and healing powers of lavender oil.

87. A mucousy discharge from (in this case) the penis.

88. Similar to a pessary but smaller, and for insertion into the urethra.

89. The title of this brochure would seem to confirm that the word "aromatherapy" was not yet in use in 1916.

90. Inflammation of the uterus.

91. Inflammation of the cervix.

92. Normal discharge from uterus following childbirth or abortion.

93. Having her first child.

94. This incident has become something of a myth. There seems little doubt that it played an important role in alerting Gattefossé to the healing powers of essential oils, and therefore may have contributed significantly to the development of aromatherapy. However, this did not herald the discovery of aromatherapy per se. The burns must have been severe to lead to gas gangrene, a very serious infection.

95. Others have, more recently, noticed a similar scenario, which may be due to a combination of antisepsis and immune stimulation. This synergy may be much more powerful *in vivo* than antisepsis *in vitro*.

96. Localised inflammation of connective tissue.

97. Glandular inflammation.

98. Joining together.

99. An offensive discharge from the nostrils due to a clinical condition.

100. Present day volatile solvent extracts, or absolutes, are not generally speaking more toxic than steam distilled oils. However, if the products used in Gattefossé's time had high levels of solvent residue, e.g. benzene, this might very well account for the higher toxicity levels he observed.

101. Accumulation of fluid.

102. The essential oils of these four plants are indeed toxic, and all except hyssop are abortifacient.

103. Here the author is attempting to make the facts support his argument, when in reality they do not. Essential oils are not all as harmless as he clearly wants to believe them to be.

104. Increasing the activity of leucocytes in defence of the body against infection. Since Gattefossé's time research has confirmed this property of many essential oils.

105. Destruction of bacteria by dissolution.

106. Nodular, vesicular.

107. Hydrated skin is now known to absorb essential oils more readily than dehydrated skin.

108. Essential oils and their major components, such as eugenol and menthol, are still widely used in dental hygiene products today.

109. The information given in this section is, understandably, very dated and much toxicological research has been conducted since. For a full update see *The Essential Oil Safety Data Manual* by R. Tisserand and T. Balacs, Brighton, 1993.

110. This was certainly true in 1937, but would not apply today.

111. Almost certainly this is untrue.

112. Whether HCN should be regarded as a mere "impurity" is debatable, since it forms a natural part of the distilled essential oil.

113. Certainly, bitter almond oil with HCN is toxic, and without is not.

114. During the earlier part of this century juniper oil was often referred to as being toxic, or abortifacient. Modern toxicological research does not support this view, which may have originated due to a confusion between "juniper" (*Juniperus communis*) and "savin" (*Juniperus sabina*) which is indeed both toxic and abortifacient.

115. There are no recent data that support Gattefossé's views regarding the dangers of juniper, pinene, turpentine, pine etc.

116. These comments may be true of savin, and other oils containing *toxic* ketones. Fennel and caraway are not currently thought to be toxic, and are widely used in food flavourings.

117. None of the five essences referred to here are regarded as toxic today.

118. This is true of safrole, which is now known to be a very mild carcinogen. Safrole is found in sassafras oil.

119. Aggregations and perhaps, therefore, deposits.

120. Gattefossé was not the first person to use essential oils therapeutically, nor was he the only one to research and write about aromatherapy in the early 20th century. However, he deserves full credit for his vision of aromatherapy as a distinct discipline with "an illustrious future".

INDEX

A

abscesses, 40, 60, 87, 91, 105, 106 *and see* sores
absinthe, 47, 104
absorption *see* cutaneous absorption
Achillea, 31, 47
acids, 12
Acorus calamus, 29
adenitis, 76, 77, 78
adenophlegmons, 92 *and see* phlegmons
African pellitory, 31
ajowan, 32
akerkarhà *see* African pellitory
alcohols, 12, 14, 43–5, 100–1 *and see* ethyl alcohol
aldehydes, 12–13, 14, 46
aloe, 103
alopecia, 73, 75
Alpinia galanga (galangal), 17, 34, 46
amber, 22, 43, 65, 68–9, 103
ambergris, 4, 6, 7
amoebic dysentery, 84 *and see* dysentery
anaesthesia, 38
analgesia, 38, 70
anethol, 13, 47, 111, 115
angelica, 15, 50, 70, 71, 85, 110
    properties, 22, 32
angina, 46, 60
animal smells, 4–8, 31
animals, treatment of *see* veterinary medicine
anise, 22, 31, 47, 111, 115
    properties, 23, 33, 116
aniseed, 46, 60, 71, 103–4 *and see* star anise
antipyogenic mixture, 58
antiseptics, viii, 44, 46, 89, 107–9, 111–12
antispasmodic mixture, 58
Apium see celery
arnica, 65
aromadendral, 41
aromadendrene, 41–2
aromatherapy, v, 56
aromatic constituents, 14–15
aromatic substances, 15–20, 71
artemisia, 47 *and see* genepi
arterial hypertension, 46, 69, 70
asafoetida, 23, 30, 69
Asarum blumei, 29
asphalt, 86

asthma, 58
Atlas cedar, 33, 73, 76, 86 *and see* cedar
atonic dyspepsia, 44, 71
atonic wounds, 76, 77, 95–6, 104–6 *and see* wounds

B
bactericides, 48
balanitis, 77
balneology, 109–10
balsamic mixture, 57
basil, 23
baths, 109–10
bay, 15, 74
bdellium, 23
beavers, 5
bedsores, 74, 106
benzoates, 45–6
benzoic aldehyde, 46 *and see* aldehydes
benzoin, 23, 30, 111
bergamot, 9, 44, 50, 84
    characteristics, 12–13, 16
    properties, 23, 33
Bijou du Dauphiné, 23–4
birch, 65
birthworts, 29
bitter almonds, 115
bitter orange, 16, 61
bleeding, 31, 47
blennorrhoea, 79
Blumea balsamifera, 29
bokhour el berber *see* ser'hin
boldo, 33
Borneo camphor, 33, 43–4 *and see* camphor
borneol, 9, 29, 33, 40, 43–5, 70
bornyl ethers, 9 *and see* ethers
bronchial spasms, 46
bronchitis, 32, 58, 64
bruising, 65
burnet, 60
burns, 87, 90–1, 95, 105
butyrates, 45–6

C
cade
    oil of, 23, 73
    balsam, 75

cajeput, 30, 33, 69, 109, 116
calamus, 17, 65, 69, 85
calciferol, 52
campanula root, 85
camphene, 44
camphor, 23, 43–4, 69, 85, 88 *and see* Borneo camphor, Japanese
    camphor
Canada balsam, 23
cancer, 72, 74, 84
caraway, 14, 16, 23, 47, 71, 115
cardamom, 16
carnation, 110
carotene, 51
carrot *see* wild carrot
carvacrol, 13, 14, 48, 112
carvone, 47
case studies, 74–80, 81–3, 90–4
castoreum, 5, 6–7, 69
catarrh, 103
cedar, 60, 71, 73, 76 *and see* Atlas cedar
cedrene, 29
cedria, 73
cedrol, 29
Cedrus atlantica, 73, 76 *and see* cedar
celery, 16, 23, 33, 110
cervicitis, 81
Ceylon cinnamon, 33 *and see* cinnamon
Ceylon citronella oil, 13, 16 *and see* citronella
chancroids, 76, 77–8, 80
chapping, 74
chiang, 46
China root (*Smilax China L.*), 30
Chinese cinnamon, 33 *and see* cinnamon
Chinese medicine, 29–30
chio turpentine, 23–4 *and see* turpentine
chios mastic, 31 *and see* mastic
chlorophyll, 51
cholera, 104
cineol, 44
cinnamic aldehyde, 112 *and see* aldehydes
cinnamon, 24, 33, 46, 103, 111
cinnamon bark, 16
cinnamon leaf, 16, 112
citral, 13, 46
citron peel, 9
citronella, 13, 16, 18

citronellol, 12, 112
civet, 7, 22,68
clary sage, 24, 45
clove, 48, 69, 74, 85, 111, 112, 116
   characteristics, 14
   properties, 24, 33
clove-cinnamon or clove-nutmeg, 24
colds, 32, 47, 58
colic, 31, 46
condylomas, 74
constipation, 46
convulsions, 7, 30
copaiba, 24, 31–2, 33, 71, 76
coriander, 47, 50, 109
   characteristics, 16–17
   properties, 24, 33
coryza, 42, 64
costus, 24
cresol, 59, 112
Crataegus oxyacantha L. (hawthorn), 69
Crotum tiglium L., 29
cubeb, 17, 76
cumin, 24
Curcuma tinctoria, 29
cutaneous absorption, 61, 62–5, 109
cypress, 33, 59, 60
cystitis, 32
cytophylactic power of essences, 104–6

D
dandruff, 73, 75
decomposition, 3
decongestant mixture, 58
delirium tremens, 7
dendemo leaves, 31
dental surgery, 48, 110–14
dermatosis, 74
diabetes mellitus, 71
diarrhoea, 31
diet, and smell, 8
digestive tract, 71–2
dill, 33
Dipterocarpus turbinatus, 76
diphtheria, 59–60, 104
disease, and smells, 7–8
disinfectants, 42, 71

dittany of Crete, 24
diuretics, 71–2, 110
dressings, 46, 87–8, 107–9
Dryobalanops, 43 *and see* borneol
dysentery, 31, 84
dysmenorrhoea, 31
dyspepsia, 44, 71
dysphagia, 60

E
earache, 22
Eberthella typhosa, 104
eczema, 74–5, 116
electromagnetic composition, 118–19
embalming, 3, 86–7
embalming of sores, 87–94
endometriosis, 82
energy, 22
epilepsy, 6, 47, 68
ergosterol, 52
essential oils, xi, 8, 10, 22–8, 32–5, 118–19
    classification, 12–20
    and dressings, 107–9
    mixing, 56
    storing, 42, 56
    terpeneless, 13–14
    therapeutic uses, 49–50
esters, 12, 45
estragole, 13
ethers, 9, 14, 45–6
ethyl alcohol, 98–104
eucalyptol, 40, 88
eucalyptus, 40, 41–2, 60, 116
    and absorption, 63
    characteristics, 17
    properties, 34
eucalyptus leaf, 71
Eucommia ulmoides, 30
eugenol, 13, 48, 83, 111, 112, 113
Euscaphis japonica, 30
expectorant mixture, 57
experimentation, 38–9, 45–6, 69, 70, 98–101, 114
eye problems, 31

F
fenchone, 47, 99
fennel, 47, 50, 71, 99, 115

characteristics, 17
properties, 34
fern, 110
fertility, 31
Ferula alliacea, 30
fever, 22, 44 *and see* rheumatic fever, scarlet fever
fibroma, 82
fir, 44, 109
fistulas, 106
fixation abscesses, 40, 87, 91 *and see* abscesses
flatulence, 30
Forgue, Dr, case studies, 80, 93–4
formols, 112
Four Thieves Vinegar, 85–6
frankincense, 72
French peppermint, 17
furunculosis, 49

G
galangal (*Alpinia galanga*), 17, 34, 46
galbanum, 24
gangrene, 64, 87, 90, 93
garlic, 85
Gattefossé, René-Maurice, v–vi, vii, 134–7
gauzes, 107
genepi (*Artemisia spicata*), 25
geraniol, 12, 13, 45, 112
geranium, 60, 84, 87, 112, 116
charcteristics, 12, 17
properties, 24, 34
ginger, 17
gingivitis, 31
ginseng (*Panax ginseng*), 29, 30
goats, odour of, 59
goat's rue, 25
gonorrhoea, 31, 32, 79 *and see* venereal diseases
guaiacol, 63, 88, 112
gummas, 77, 80
gums (mouth), 31
gurjun balsam, 76, 86
gynaecology, 80–3

H
Haemophylus ducreyi, 77, 78
haemorrhoids, 47, 84
hawthorn (*Crataegus oxyacantha L.*), 69

headaches, 7, 22, 31–2
heart, 7, 22, 30, 46, 69–70
helichrysum, 25
heliotrope, 69
herbal wines, 103
hiccups, 46
horehound, 85
hormones, 7, 10
human smells, vii–viii, 2–3, 7–8
hydrocyanic acid, 115
hyssop, 61, 74. 84, 103, 104, 109
    characteristics, 17–18
hysteria, 7, 68–9

I
incense, 86
influenza, 42, 83–4
inhalations, 57–9, 62
injections, 38–9, 62, 87
insects, smells, viii, 4–5
intestinal diseases, 103
Inula helenium L., 59
iodine, 77
iris, 25

J
Japanese camphor, 34, 43, 70 *and see* camphor
jasmine, 25, 110
Java citronella, 13, 18 *and see* citronella
juniper, 44, 50, 65, 71, 74, 115
    characteristics, 18
    properties, 25, 34
Juniperus chinensis, 29
Juniperus oxycedrus, 73

K
kayaputi *see* cajeput
ketones, 12, 14, 47, 115
kidney vetch, 25
kidneys, 71–2

L
lactones, 14, 15
ladanum (labdanum), 25, 31
laryngitis, 7
laurel waters, 69
Laurus camphora, 30
lavender, 22, 49, 65, 82, 84, 87, 105
    case studies, 74–80, 82, 90–6

characteristics, 12–13, 18
    in dentistry, 113
    for embalming, 86, 87
    properties, 25, 34, 44, 45
lavender stoechas, 25
lemon, 9, 50, 115
    characteristics, 13–14, 18
    properties, 25, 34
lemongrass, 13–14, 50
lentisk resin, 31
leprosy, 31, 74
lesions, 90, 95
light, ix, 10
lilac, 110
lime, 14, 18
limonene, 13, 40
linalol, 44–5
linalyl acetate, 13
liqueurs, 47, 100–1, 102–4
liquidambar, 25
liver cancer, 84
lovage, 71, 110
lycopene, 51, 52

mace, 65
Magnolia denudata, 30
malaria, 42, 44, 103
Mallotus philippinensis, 29–30
mandarin, 18
Marchand, Dr, case studies, 75–9, 90–1
marjoram, 85
Marseille vinegar, 85
massage, 65
mastic, 26, 31, 86
masticatories, 71, 73
matico essence, 76
meadowsweet, 85
measles, 64
Melaleuca alternifolia (tea tree), 32
melissa, 26, 69
meningococcus, 104
menthol, 14, 35, 111
menthone, 47, 49–50
metacresyl phenylacetate, 59
methyl anthranilate, 69
methylheptenone, 13

metritis, 81, 82
Meurisse, Dr, case studies, 74–5, 79, 80–3, 91–3, 94
minerals, smells, 10
mint, 46, 47, 49–50, 60, 111
    characteristics, 14
    properties, 26, 34
mint water, 69
mirbane, essence of, 114
miscarriage, 81
molluscs, smells, 4
mouth ulcers, 31, 60
mouthwashes, 59–60, 111, 113–14
mummification, 3 *and see* embalming
mumps, 64
musk, 6, 7, 22, 68, 69, 103
musk deer, 6
musk octopus, 4
myristicin, 116
myrrh, 103
myrtle, 69

N
narcosis, 66–8
narcotics, 70
natron, 86
neroli, 34, 69
nerve balsam/ointment, 74
nervous centres, 68–70
nitrobenzene, 114
Norwegian pine, 18 *and see* pine
nutmeg butter, 74

O
obstetrics, 80–3
ointments, 64–5, 74, 107–8
olibanum, 72
olive oil, 48, 84
onyx, 4
operation pneumonia, 66
opopanax, 26
orange, 9, 14, 50
orangeflower, 44, 69, 115
oregano, 72, 109
origanum, 26
osteitis, 94
otitis, 64

ovaries, 30
oxides, 14
ozaena, 94
ozone, 41–2

P
paenol, 29
Paeonia moutan, 29
palpitations, 7
panacene, 29
Panax ginseng (ginseng), 29, 30
Panax repens (tam-thât), 30
parsley, 71, 110
pennyroyal, 26
peppermint, 17
Peru balsam, 26, 73, 88
petitgrain, 18, 50
petroleum jelly, 88
phagedenas, 48, 76
pharmacopoeias, 29
phellandrene, 41–2
Phellodendron, 30
phenols, 12–13, 14, 15, 48–9, 83, 88, 111–12, 115
phlegmons, 91, 105 *and see* adenophlegmons
phytol, 51–2
pimenta leaf, 18–19
pine, 18, 19, 26, 40, 44, 83, 87, 109
pinene, 41–2, 44, 115
piperitone, 41, 42
pityriasis, 73–4, 75
plague, 6, 43, 44, 84–6
plant smells, viii, 8–10
pleurisy, 46
pneumonia, 64, 66
Pomatum muscitae compositum, 74
Popowia capea, 31
pruritus, 74, 82
psoriasis, 73
puerperal infections, 81
pulmonary ailments, 61–4
pyramidon, 82
pyrethrum root, 111

Q
quai sun, 31
quinine, 84

R

ramangoaka root, 31
rambiazana, 31
religion, and smells, 3, 29
respiratory tract, 30, 48, 57–61
revulsion, 61–8
rhatany, 111
rheumatic fever, 7
rheumatic pain, 31, 76, 109
rhodium wood, 26
ringworm, 73
rose, 22, 26, 34, 69, 110, 112
rosemary, 44, 65, 71, 74, 85, 103
    characteristics, 19
    properties, 34
rosewater, 8, 69
rue, 26–7, 65, 85, 104

S

safrole, 29, 116
sage, 22, 30, 44, 60, 69, 74, 85, 103
    characteristics, 19
    properties, 27, 35
Salies de Béarn salts, 82
Salvol, 79, 80–2, 83, 89
salvone, 79
sandalwood, 71, 76, 110
Sapolinol, 84, 89, 105
sassafras, 19, 27, 109, 110
Sassard, Dr P., case studies, 95–6, 106
savin, 27, 65, 115
savory, 22, 27, 70
scabies, 73
scarlet fever, 64
sciatica, 103
Scots pine, 19 *and see* pine
scrofula, 74
seborrhoea, 73
sedatives, 57, 70
septicaemia, 43
ser'hin/sarhina, 30–1
sesquiterpenes, 15, 76
sex, and smells, 3, 4–5, 68
Siberian pine, 87 *and see* pine
siccative mixture, 58
skin, 49, 52, 72–4, 116

and revulsion, 62–3, 65
smells, vii, xi–xii
  animal, 4–8, 31
  and diet, 8
  and disease, 7–8
  human, vii–viii, 2–3, 7–8
  insects, viii, 4–5
  minerals, 10
  molluscs, 4
  onyx, 4
  plants, viii, 8–10
  and religion, 3, 29
  and sex, 3, 4–5, 68
Smilax China L. (China root), 30
smoking, 72
sodium cinnamate, 60
solubility, 50
sores, 31, 47, 48, 73, 77, 90–1, 95–6
  embalming of, 87–94
  and see abscesses
sperm whales, 6
spike lavender, 49 *and see* lavender
spruce, 109
staphylococcus, 104
star anise, 19, 27, 35, 47, 60, 116 *and see* aniseed
sterols, 52
stimulants, 7
stomach problems, 22, 31, 46, 50, 103
styrax, 27, 86
surgery, 64
sweet orange, 19
syphilis, 78–9, 80 *and see* venereal diseases

T
tam-thât (*Panax repens*), 30
tansy, 27, 70, 104
tasserr'int/tausserghimt *see* ser'hin
tea tree (*Melaleuca alternifolia*), 32
terpeneless essences, 13–14, 50, 56
terpenes, 9–10, 12–13, 14, 15, 20, 39–40, 115
  inhalations, 58–9
terpineol, 9, 40, 44–5
tetanus, 7, 31–2
throat infections, 60
thuja, 74
thujone, 47, 70, 116

thyme, 48, 59, 65, 72, 74, 86
   characteristics, 14, 19
   properties, 27, 35
   and see wild thyme
thymol, viii, 13, 14, 48, 83, 112
   and absorption, 63
   properties, 35
tikentest *see* African pellitory
tobacco, 72
tolu, balsam of, 23
toothache, 6, 22, 47
toothpastes, 31, 46, 111
toxicity, 40, 53, 70, 98–104, 114–16
tracheitis, 64
tranquillisers, 69
treponemas, 78
trioxymethylene, 112
tsianiamposa wood, 31
tsiborata root, 31
tuberculosis, 59, 60, 64
tulle gras, 107
Turkey red oil, 79
turpentine, 9, 40, 49, 60, 65, 86, 109–10, 115 *and see* chio turpentine
typhoid, 7

U
ulcers
   digestive tract, 72
   mouth, 31, 60
   skin, 95, 106
   stomach, 46, 50
   varicose, 94
Umbelliferae, 30
uterus, 30

V
vaginitis, 79
valerian, 27, 69
valuvy root, 31
vanilla, 28, 69
vanillin, 116
varicose ulcers, 94
venereal diseases, 75–7 *and see* gonorrhoea, syphilis
verbena, 28
veterinary medicine, 43, 49, 74, 83
violet, 110

vitamins, 51–3
voanana leaves, 31
voaseya leaves, 31
vomiting, 31, 60
vulnerary mixture, 58

W
warts, 74
whitlows, 105
whooping cough, 7, 46, 58, 59
wild carrot, 28
wild celery *see* celery
wild thyme, 28, 64 *and see* thyme
wines, 103 *and see* liqueurs
wintergreen, 65
wormwood, 22, 47, 85, 104, 115
   characteristics, 20
   properties, 28, 35
wounds, 90, 92–3
   atonic, 76, 77, 95–6, 104–6

X
xanthophyll, 51

Y
yarrow, 28, 35, 47

Z
zana bark, 31
zinc eugenate, 113
zinc oxide, 113
zit ou zâäter, 48